Tales of the Exam Room Volume 6**: Heartbreaking Medical Stories**

This is a work of fiction. Unless otherwise stated – all names, characters, businesses, places, events, locales, and incidents in this book are the product of either the author's imagination or are used in a fictitious manner. Any resemblance to actual persons, living or dead, or actual events is purely coincidental.

ISBN: 978-1-954814-65-3 (Paperback)

ISBN: 978-1-954814-64-6 (EBook)

First Edition 2023.

Credits:

Book Cover and Formatting by: farhanshahid101

Obsidian Wolf Publishing

PO Box 1086 Salem, UT 84653

Contents

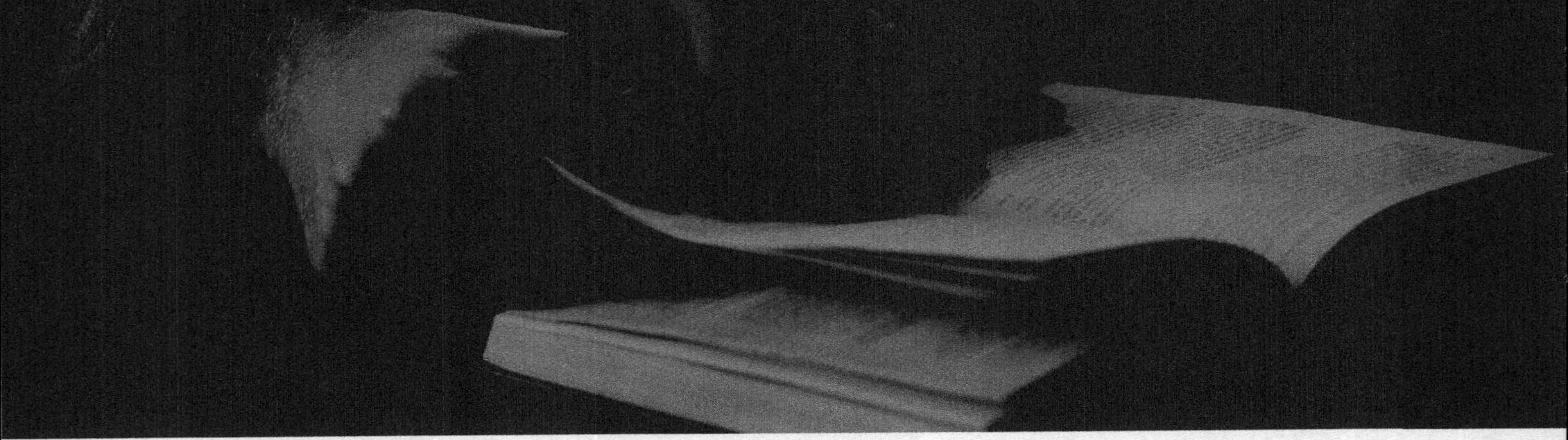

Introduction

This is Volume 6 of Tales of the Exam Room: Heartbreaking Medical Stories

These tales are intended to be felt, enjoyed, and told repeatedly. There is so much to learn about patient encounters, decision-making disasters, and the incredible actions of those involved during odd and life-saving situations.

Whether you come to this book having read the last five and enjoy our stories, or you are new to the wild world of crazy medical stories, we hope that you will enjoy this volume. If this is your first time, please check out our other four volumes.

This is our 6th volume, and we will focus on examining the difficult sides of medicine, treatment, and circumstances. Many patients want the best possible outcome, and so do their families and friends. Unfortunately, that is not always in the cards. That doesn't mean these stories all have depressing outcomes, but heartbreak is a common theme.

Author Scott Kemp brings his latest short story collection with the hopes that you will feel the pain and discomfort the patient may be experiencing and learn from it.

Additionally, it is important to understand that individuals may make decisions about future treatment and prognosis based on their fears or misunderstandings about what medicine may or may not provide for them. You might think you might act differently, but it would be hard to understand unless you were walking in their shoes truly.

Remember that the art of medicine is seldom straightforward and common sense is not always common.

Please Enjoy and Feel Free to Join Us for additional medical stories @examroomtales.com.

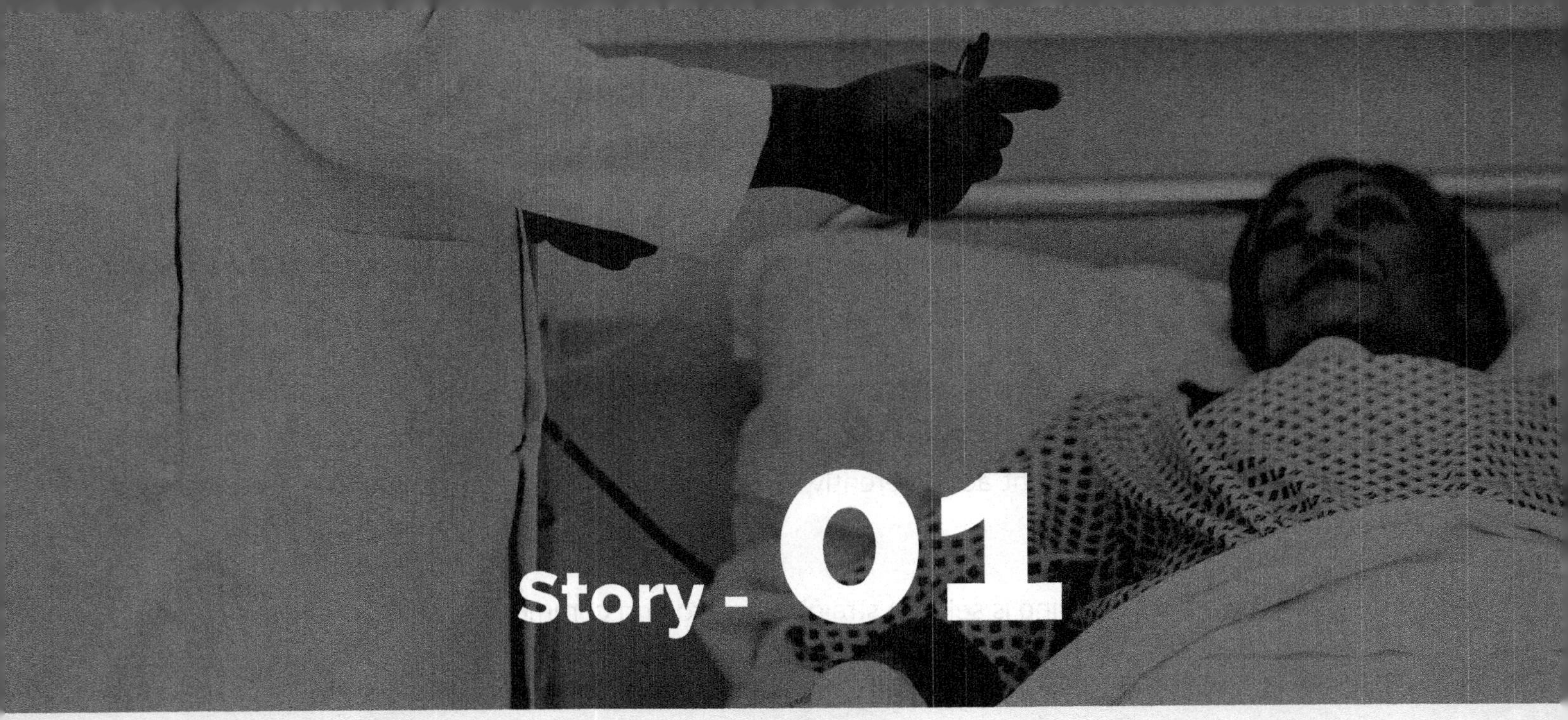

Chronic Chest and Abdominal Pain that Just Won't Go Away.

Florence walked into the Emergency Room feeling the worst she had felt in two or three weeks. It was nearly four in the morning, but a half dozen people were waiting to be brought back into a room. Florence was upset and unsure that going to the doctor again was the right thing to do. This was her fourth visit to see someone, and she didn't think she would get any more answers.

The first two times, she had seen her regular doctor, who gave her some things to look for, dietary changes, and some medications. Those recommendations worked for about six months, but then her symptoms returned. The last time she came to the ER, she left with no answers and more questions.

An hour ago, she woke from a dead sleep with chest and abdominal pain that was on a whole new level. It was far worse than when she had come to the hospital previously. She had blood work done, received an EKG, and was given an IV and some medications. The doctor explained that it hadn't been a heart attack and thought it might be a muscle spasm or some heartburn.

Florence could not help herself and gave a gigantic eye roll.

Heartburn had been what her primary care physician had said as well, over ten months ago. She had been given two medications to help treat the symptoms. They had sort of worked for six months. She and her husband had started exercising a bit more, and she had lost ten pounds. She avoided certain foods that seemed to make things work and explicitly avoided eating after eight p.m.

"Can I help you?" asked the receptionist.

"I'm having chest and abdominal pain that started an hour ago. This is the worst it has ever been."

"Have you been seen for this before?"

"A few times, but it isn't getting any better."

"Who have you seen?"

"I came to this ER about three weeks ago. Before that, I saw my doctor. I explained all of this the last time I was here."

"I see."

Florence spent the next ten minutes working out insurance issues and paying a copay.

"Have a seat, and we'll call you back as soon as possible."

"Thank you," Florence said, turning to find where her husband was sitting. He had parked the car when she had come in.

When she sat down, he said, "The billboard shows a fifteen-minute wait."

"I think it will be longer than that."

Nurse Dawn brought her back to her room an hour later. This lady was older, kind, and talkative. Florence learned a lot about the women even before she was settled in her room. Her blood pressure was normal, 133/79. All her vitals were normal as well.

"Does that mean anything?" Florence asked.

"Maybe." Nurse Dawn added, "I think that Dr. Bradly will want an EKG. Have you ever had one before?"

"A few different times. I was here three weeks ago with the same complaint. It is much worse this time. They did an EKG at the time and some blood work."

"Oh great," Nurse Dawn said. "We can pull that one up and compare it to today's."

"Okay."

"What about medications?"

"I take some for anxiety, depression, thyroid, and two for gastric reflux disease."

"Thanks. I'll go talk to the doctor and be back in a few minutes."

Nurse Dawn was gone for fifteen minutes. When she returned, she said, "He does want some blood work, an IV, an EKG, and some medicine that you can drink."

"I remember that. It didn't taste very good the last time."

Nurse Dawn smiled. "It doesn't taste any better. You would think that after all this time, they could come up with a better-tasting combination."

"I wish." Florence got undressed, and the pads were placed on her chest. It took five minutes to get everything with the EKG done.

Nurse Dawn said, "We have a newer nurse who would like to come in and start your IV. Is that acceptable?"

Florence shrugged.

A tall man, nearly six feet two, came in. His hands were big, but he was gentle. He was introduced as Eric. He did a wonderful job, and on the first try, he expertly placed the IV. Blood was first taken out to be sent off, and some fluids were started. Last, the cocktail of liquids was given, and she downed the entire shot.

Twenty minutes later, Dr. Bradly arrived holding a chart. He introduced himself and dove right in. "I read the report from the last time you were here. The EKG from last time and this time look the same. We'll wait for the lab results, but it doesn't appear to be cardiac."

"That's not the news I was hoping for."

"Really?"

"I want to understand what is causing this. It is miserable. I can't begin to describe how horrible I feel."

"Are you feeling any better after the concoction that you drank?"

"A little?"

"Have you ever had a colonoscopy or an endoscopy?"

"Which one goes into your intestines?"

"The colonoscopy."

"I had that a few years ago. I've never had the other."

"Sometimes when a patient has heartburn that is not well controlled by the medications they are taking, it might be important to get a camera into the stomach to see if there are ulcers or other things."

"Can I have that done here?"

"No. But we will schedule you an appointment and can get it done in the next week."

Florence felt a small amount of relief for the first time in a long time.

"There is also a test to check for a certain bacteria in the stomach called H. pylori. We will test for that as well," replied Dr. Bradly.

"Did they check for that the last time?"

"I don't think so. Previously, they were focused on the heart because that was where most of your pain was. However, this is the second time we've seen you, and it sounds like your primary provider has seen you a few times. Seeing a gastro specialist is the next step. Can I do an exam?"

Florence nodded.

The exam was detailed, and Florence was relieved that Dr. Bradley took the time to check her out. Once he was finished, he asked, "Have you had any weight loss, night sweats, nausea, loss of appetite, or anything else?"

"My doctor recommended that we change our diet and increase our exercise. He said that some heartburn could be related to being slightly overweight. My husband and I are healthy, but we have worked hard. I think I've lost ten pounds. I don't eat as much as I used to, and I am past having hot flashes with menopause."

"That's good to hear. Why don't you relax and we'll wait for the results of your labs. It shouldn't be much longer. If everything turns out normal and you are feeling better, we will probably let you go home."

Florence said, "Thank you."

When the doctor left, Florence's husband asked, "Are you feeling any better?"

"A little."

Thirty minutes later, Nurse Dawn and Dr. Bradley came into the room. Dr. Bradley said, "Everything came back normal. Looks like you are in good health. I've written you a referral to get an endoscopy next week. They will call with the directions and where you need to go."

"Okay."

"I've also increased your proton-pump inhibitor. The medication you take for your stomach. It will still be twice a day, but the dose is increased."

"If you say so."

Nurse Dawn said, "Are you feeling any better?"

"The drink helped a tiny bit for like twenty minutes. Now, I feel as bad as ever."

"Where is the pain?" asked Dr. Bradley, and he stepped closer.

Florence pointed to her stomach, her chest, and even her back. "It feels like someone is stabbing me."

Dr. Bradley said, "Let's get her set up for a chest and abdominal CT. Everything else has been normal, but I want to make sure we aren't missing anything."

Florence was pushed to the back fifteen minutes later. When she returned, Florence was in bad shape. The pain was far worse than ever. Luckily, the nurse had gotten orders to give some pain medications. When the medication finally started helping, Florence felt the first sense of pain relief in weeks. She had not realized how much pain she had been in.

Dr. Bradley came in sometime later, and he was pale and unsteady.

Florence's husband asked, "What is wrong? Did you find something?"

"We did. I think we know what is causing your pain."

"Is it bad?"

He nodded his head. "The CT of your chest and abdomen shows that you have a large pancreatic tumor. All indications show that it has moved to some of the surrounding tissue. You will be admitted tonight and will see oncology tomorrow."

"Oh, my lord. Finally."

"What do you mean finally?" asked Dr. Bradley.

"Now I finally know this pain is not all in my head."

"It's definitely not. But this is going to be a long and difficult road."

"I've lived a good life," said Florence. "But I'm not ready to give up yet. I'm ready for whatever comes."

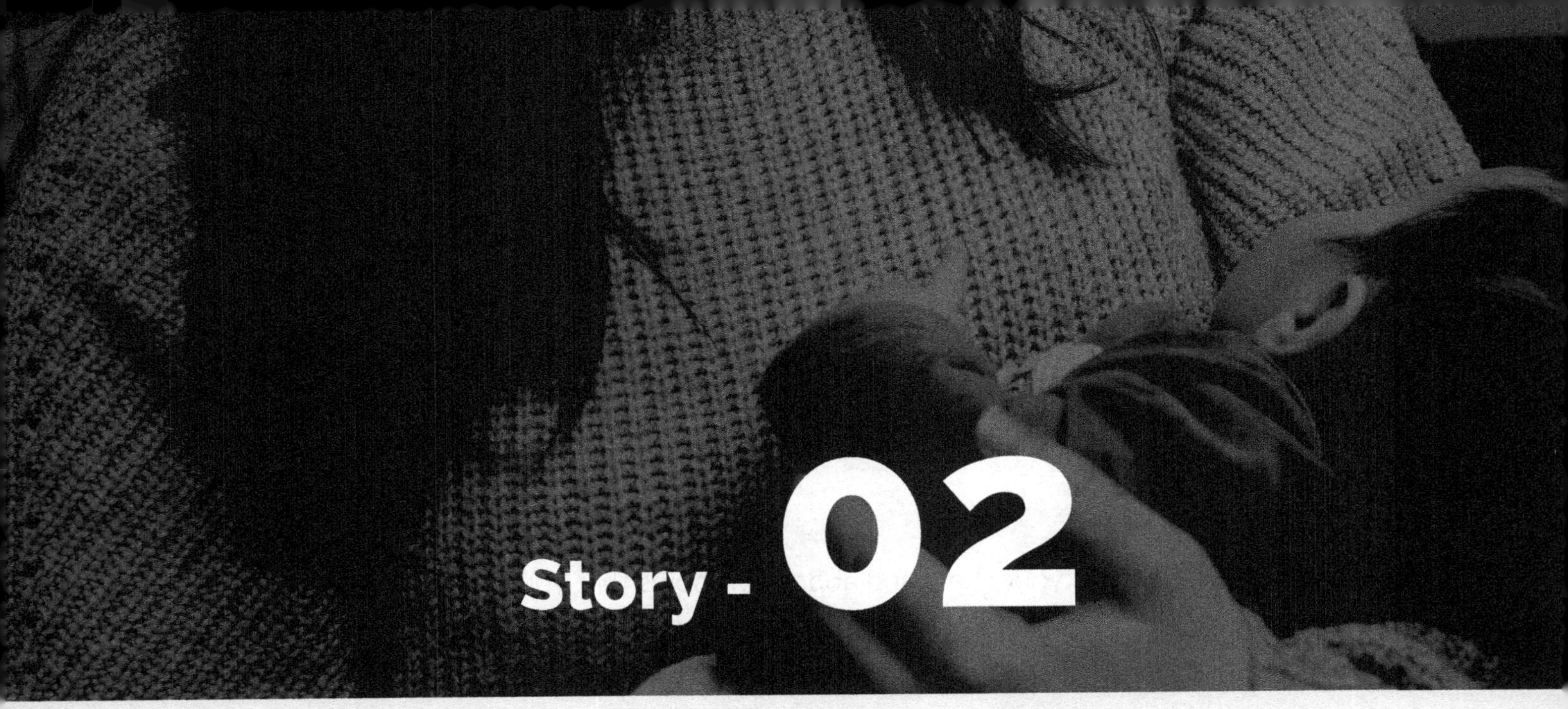

Story - 02

Milk is Good for the Body...Mostly

Dr. Gabriel was excited to see his next patient of the day. Jessica Hampton had been a young child when he first opened his practice. As she grew, he saw her often, and now she was married with four children. He was excited to see her and her family over the years, and today was no exception. It had been about six months since she had last been in his office, and if he remembered correctly, a lot had changed in her life.

There was a strange smell of decay and sickness as Dr. Gabriel opened the door, and he was worried he would find someone with a serious infection or illness. Jessica sat on the exam table, appearing miserable, pale, and uncomfortable. She had a box of Kleenex and was actively trying to prevent a sneeze.

He wondered if she had lost some weight and checked the chart. She had lost fifteen pounds since his last visit. Dr. Gabriel said, "Mrs. Hampton, it's good to see you, but it seems that you aren't feeling well. How are things?"

"Oh, Dr. Gabriel, it seems like I might be coming down with something. This is the third or fourth time in the last two months. No matter what I do, I just can't seem to stay healthy. I had a cold, a sinus problem, diarrhea for a few weeks, and now another cold."

"How bad has it been? What kind of symptoms have you had?"

"I've had with energy and sleeping. I don't have the energy to keep the house clean and only make dinner three times a week. All I want to do is sleep but I can never fall asleep. I had bad stomach cramping and a few times I had hives all over my body. When I had diarrhea, I was taking over-the-counter medications all the time."

"That sounds like the worst."

"It was." A small smile crossed her face. "Things have been so much harder with our last child. I keep thinking that it will get easier, but it doesn't."

"How is ...?"

"...Jack," Jessica finished. "He's good, but he has been much more challenging than my other kids. Obviously, I don't feel great, but he has been sicker than my other kids. I'm really here to bounce a few things off of you about him."

"What's going on?"

"He is fussy. He'll be super hungry, eat, but then he won't eat for a few days. He spits up a lot. I've started to think he might have some food allergies. Even my older kids have trouble eating some foods. They are all much pickier with foods, and honestly meals just don't sit well with any of us. I have my own stresses and trouble sleeping. My husband recommended I come to see you."

"I'm glad that you did," said Dr. Gabriel. "When did this all start?"

"Months ago. Even before we came home from the hospital with Jack."

"How old is Jack now?"

"About eight months."

"And you think he has some food allergies, or could it be something else?"

"All I can think of is an allergy. We have no new pets, haven't moved, or anything else out of the ordinary. We tried to introduce foods like vegetables, apples, and pears slowly. He doesn't handle these types of foods very well."

"Does he get rashes, become flushed, stomach aches, or anything else?"

"Jack coughs a lot and like I said, he spit up everything we gave him. I wish he wouldn't keep the food down better."

"What does your pediatrician think?"

Jessica stared at her feet. "We haven't told him yet. He doesn't really get our family. He's a nice guy and all, but he' s somewhat unusual. He doesn't listen to what I am saying and is always in his computer. He wants us to come back every few months and get shots and check-ups. He is really a by-the-books type of person."

"I see." Dr. Gabriel pulled up a chair and sat down. "When did you start with baby foods?"

"We don't use baby foods. We've heard that those foods aren't organic enough, and much of the nutritional value has been lost. We puree most everything ourselves or our neighbor does. Jack really loves milk."

"When did he start drinking milk?"

"When Jack was about four months."

Dr. Gabriel nodded. "No judgement here, but did you try to breastfeed Jack?"

"Yes. I tried. A close friend said I shouldn't get him fixated on the milk coming from me. It won't be around forever. We started supplementing with regular milk and we heard formula is poorly prepared."

Dr. Gabriel was slightly surprised by these last few statements. He knew Jessica rather well, and he remembered her other children. He didn't think she had these opinions the last time he'd seen her. He also knew that this was a sensitive topic. Telling someone to change their diet is always a tough thing to do. He said, "There are some basic guidelines on when new foods should be introduced and when to use cows' milk. Have you looked up this data?"

"My best friend, she's also my neighbor, thinks that the guidelines are just suggestions. She has shown me a lot of literature that says that for a smarter and more independent child, you need to push them a little and give them new stimulation, like unusual foods, situations, and types of learning. She told me that she gave her children regular milk, and they all turned out fine."

"I'm all for helping children find avenues to advance, but what you're suggesting with regard to food isn't the case. New foods need to be added slowly and at the right time. Allergies are something that can be concerning for any child. I don't think you should worry too much about overdoing breast milk or formula. That should be the foundation of their nutrition. The added food should be to introduce them to new things and see what they like."

"If you think so," Jessica said, and there was a clear change in her countenance like she didn't agree with his thought process.

"Is Jack here?"

"No. He's with my neighbor."

"Do you know how his weight has been?"

"I don't think he has gained any weight the last few months. I wish he was more active."

"I see." Dr. Gabriel paused for a moment. After some thought, he said, "Jessica. I've seen you for years. I'm just trying to help. We see a lot of children come in through these doors. I would love for you to make some changes and see what happens."

"That's why I'm here."

"Why don't we start with some simple food changes? What does your husband think?"

"He and I have different opinions. We've argued about it constantly. He let me try my way for a few months, and I promised him that I would talk with you. I might not agree with you completely, but I'm willing to try."

"Terrific. Let's have you go back to breastfeeding as much as possible, along with formula, if it becomes a problem. The introduction of foods needs to be slow. So, let's do nothing for one week. Then we can pick some puree foods, baby foods, like peas or squash, and one fruit. Give this to him for another week or so and see how he does. I want to see both of you back in the clinic in two weeks."

"If you think this will work," Jessica said, clearly resigned. She added, "Kathy, my best friend, is not going to be happy. She's the one that gives us some of the puree foods and lots of milk. Our family can't seem to get enough milk. We drink it all the time. Kathy insists that the government is trying to suppress the community by having the parents raise unprepared children."

"I totally understand. And to a certain point, I agree with her. But if you are sick and Jack is sick. We need to get to the bottom of things."

"I can try."

"How long has Kathy lived in the neighborhood?"

"A year. She is so sweet. She really likes us and brings us goodies all the time. She is into raising her own chickens, cows, and other animals. She produced much of her own foods, and she loves growing her own vegetables. She is self-sufficient. When the kids are old enough, we are going to send them over to learn to take care of the animals."

"It really sounds like it. Does she happen to give you milk?"

"She has her own cows. She gives us a few bottles every week."

"Does she pasteurize her milk?"

"Does she what?"

"Raw milk can be harmful to humans if not done correctly. I drink raw milk from time to time, but it must come from a reputable location. Babies and children should avoid raw milk at all costs, especially Jack."

A confused look crossed Jessica's face. She mumbled, "Kathy insists that raw milk is good for babies."

"It's not. You pasteurize milk to get all the bacteria from it. This makes it safe. Though, if you get a good farm, they can keep raw milk safe, but not for babies. I think this might be your problem. Let's do some blood tests and see if we can find out why you are sick."

Jessica had several tests performed, and once she was finished, she left with a promise to make changes in their diet for two weeks and come back. She returned with Jack two weeks later, along with her husband and her other children. She was remarkably better. Turns out, Kathy was not keeping her milk or her cows very clean. The health department was called, and they came out to her house and did an investigation. Several kids and adults in the neighborhood were also sick. They called it an outbreak, and it turned out to be a pretty big deal.

Jack improved after just a few weeks of proper nutrition. His body reacted well to the balanced nutrition, and he immediately started to gain weight. His stomach issues, rashes, and everything else cleared up to normal. He gained energy, which was a good thing.

Jessica's health improved dramatically as well. She had a urinary tract infection and stomach issues, and her blood work was abnormal. Luckily it was easily treated and significantly improved when they stopped drinking unpasteurized milk.

***Raw milk is often considered quite healthy, and the choice of thousands, and when the process allows for proper collection and storage, raw milk can provide some health benefits. This story was not to discourage unpasteurized milk in the slightest but to bring awareness to the proper process.

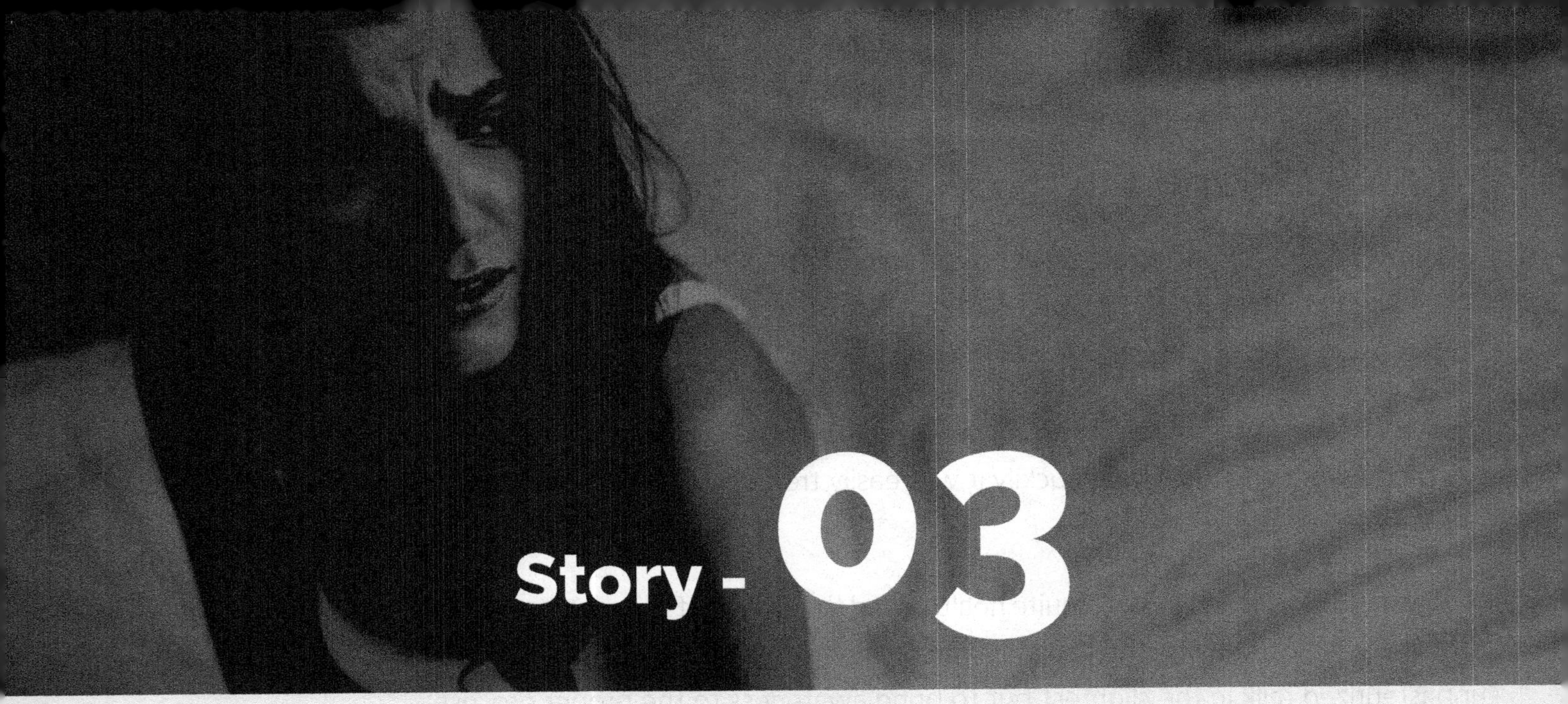

Uncomfortable Rectal Pain that Comes and Goes

Richard Hampton felt rectal pain on and off for weeks. He first thought it was hemorrhoids, then constipation, and then something popped and drained. He didn't think he had any outstanding medical problems. He hadn't been worried about the occasional blood he'd seen after wiping. He talked with a few family members and a close friend, and the consensus was that he had hemorrhoids.

He researched the internet and discovered some options he could do on his own. He made it a goal to eat more fiber, drink more water, and avoid pushing too hard. He bought some steroid cream from Walmart. The first week, there was no change, but slowly the itching and burning pain went away, and the blood could no longer be seen on the toilet paper after he used the restroom.

Additional benefits were Richard felt better, lost some weight, and had less bloating. Every third or fourth day, though, he would get some rectal pain that almost put him on his knees. He didn't understand what was happening but chalked it up to hemorrhoids.

Two weeks later, while driving home, he had had pain throughout the day. He didn't feel that a hemorrhoid was his problem, and the pain was slightly up farther up the backside rather than between his legs. He had felt a small lump and worried about what it could be. He couldn't see anything in the mirror and wanted to wait until his partner could look at the area.

Ten minutes from home, he turned a corner and felt a pop in his pants. Suddenly there was a gush of liquid in his underwear and a noticeable smell. It didn't smell good. Richard worried he had an infection. The pain or discomfort he'd felt throughout the day was gone instantly.

When he got home, he ran to his bathroom, showered, and changed his clothing. He felt around the rectal opening and didn't feel a lump, and he had no bleeding. He couldn't identify where the liquid that had stained his underwear had come from. He felt around, but there was only minimal pain and no obvious infection. He decided not to tell his partner.

Time passed, and he forgot about the incident. Six months later, he woke up and felt some rectal discomfort. He had slipped a little on his improved health regimen, and the night before, he had some constipation. It had taken thirty minutes to finally have a bowel movement. Instead of relieving him, he went to bed in pain. The pain was worse this morning, and he had significant bloating and felt sick in his stomach.

He drank some liquid fiber supplements and went to work. Around noon, he started having some fever and chills. By two o'clock, he could barely sit down. He was having a large amount of bright red blood by this point. The pain and the pressure in his backside had tripled from earlier. He felt nauseous and had no choice but to go home.

As he left his office, he called his partner, and they suggested he stop by Urgent Care. "This has been a problem long enough," they said. Richard agreed and stopped at a building ten minutes from his house.

"How can I help you?" asked the front desk receptionist.

"Stomach issues. Fever and chills, and I became nauseous a few hours ago. It's getting worse and worse."

The information was written down. Richard answered some additional questions on a form and was slightly more forthcoming. Insurance issues were settled.

Forty-five minutes later, he was called out by a nurse who asked the same questions as the front desk receptionist. He was weighed, his temperature taken, and other vitals were done. He had a temperature of 101.9 and a slightly elevated blood pressure.

Because of the temperature, he was tested for COVID, given a mask, and placed in an exam room. Twenty minutes later, the doctor came in.

Doctor Shamo said, "The nurse tells me you have some flu-like symptoms, with fever, chills, nausea, and a temperature."

"I don't think it is the flu," said Richard. "I don't have sinus issues, cough, or nasal congestion. But I am having a lot of rectal pain."

"Okay." Doctor Shamo sat in his chair. "Can you tell me more?"

"I have some on and off again constipation. I take fiber but haven't taken any in a few weeks. I felt plugged up last night, and it took a while to have a bowel movement. This morning, I didn't feel any better. I took a large amount of fiber and went to work. I started feeling sicker around noon, and I noticed blood again around 2 pm. Add in some hot and cold flashes, along with nausea, and I came here."

"When you say blood again, what does that mean?"

"I think I have hemorrhoids. I've had blood on the toilet paper before. That's when I started taking fiber more frequently. I also bought some steroid cream."

"Did that help?"

"Yes. The blood went away."

"Have you had any other symptoms?"

"Not really. I just feel really sick, and there's a lot of pressure when I sit."

"How old are you?"

"Forty-nine," Richard said.

"Have you ever had a colonoscopy?"

Richard shook his head. "I don't think so."

Doctor Shamo leaned in closer. "It's when they give you something to drink or some pills, and you use the restroom a lot. Then the next day, they knock you out and put a scope into your rectum."

"Nope," said Richard. "Never had that experience, and I really don't want to."

"It's a common concern. But, when we talk about blood in the stool in an older man or woman, we first think of something in the intestines. It's recommended for those older than forty-five."

"I don't know."

Doctor Shamo continued, "Is the blood bright red or a darker color?"

"Bright red."

"Have you ever seen blood within your stool?"

"I've never looked that hard."

"Any history of stomach ulcers?"

"Not that I am aware of."

Doctor Shamo sat back. "Any drainage, infection, or other problems."

Richard thought for a moment. Until this moment, he had forgotten about the episode in his car. He couldn't recall if what he was feeling now was similar to back then. He wasn't sure he wanted to tell the doctor about that last episode. In the end, he said, "More than six months ago, I had this tremendous pain close to my rectum. I thought I had an infection, but as I was driving home, something popped, and the pain disappeared."

"Interesting," said Doctor Shamo. "Was it a cyst or something? Did a hemorrhoid burst?"

"Can they?"

"If they're bad enough. But it's unlikely."

"The discharge got into my underwear, and it smelled really bad. I couldn't find where the boil popped if it was a cyst."

Doctor Shamo stood. "It's time for an exam."

"What kind?"

Doctor Shamo pulled on some gloves and pulled out a packet of petroleum jelly. "First, I will look at the rectal opening to see if I can see any hemorrhoids. I will check the prostate next and see if I can find any other problems."

Richard said nothing but nodded. A moment later, he pulled down his pants and underwear. He checked the rectal opening. He placed his hand on the upper portion of the buttocks, and Richard felt a jolt of pain descending to his rectum. "Ouch," he cried.

Doctor Shamo pushed the area again, and the same pain returned. He pulled open the crack and said, "I think I know part of the problem."

Richard asked, "I don't think I can handle any fingers in my rectum at present."

"I completely understand," said Doctor Shamo, and he stepped away and pulled off his gloves.

"Is that it?" asked Richard.

"Not entirely," said Doctor Shamo, and he sat back on his chair. Richard pulled up his pants and sat down as well.

"What's wrong? Do I need to take an antibiotic?"

"Eventually, you will."

"That doesn't sound horrible."

"Mr. Hampton. You have a severe case of what we call a Pilonidal Cyst."

"A cyst," interrupted Richard.

"Yes. I've seen this several times, but you have a significant one. There is an area at the top of the buttock crease that can have such a cyst. Sometimes these are overlooked because of their location. However, when they get worse, the skin in that area can be firm, raised, and red. That's what I am seeing in your case."

"And antibiotics will treat this."

"It actually needs to be cut open. We'll need to do this here. We will numb up the area as best as possible. Usually, we get a lot of drainage, and it smells terrible."

"Are you serious?"

Doctor Shamo nodded.

An hour later, Richard was finished. The entire experience was horrifying. The medication used to numb the area only partially worked. The amount of drainage was staggering. In addition, Dr. Shamo found a ball of hair, and a cup or two of drainage. Dr. Shamo said that in other cases, they had found pieces of teeth, but he'd never seen any. It was usually drainage and hair.

Richard was placed on antibiotics for a few weeks. He had a huge bandage on his buttocks. He felt dizzy for several minutes after the procedure. His symptoms would resolved, but he was warned that he might be in pain for several days after the procedure. He was extremely embarrassed. He was told this had nothing to do with cleanliness but he wasn't so sure.

As he walked out of the Urgent care, Dr. Shamo said, "Don't forget about getting your colonoscopy in the near future."

"Yeah, right," said Richard.

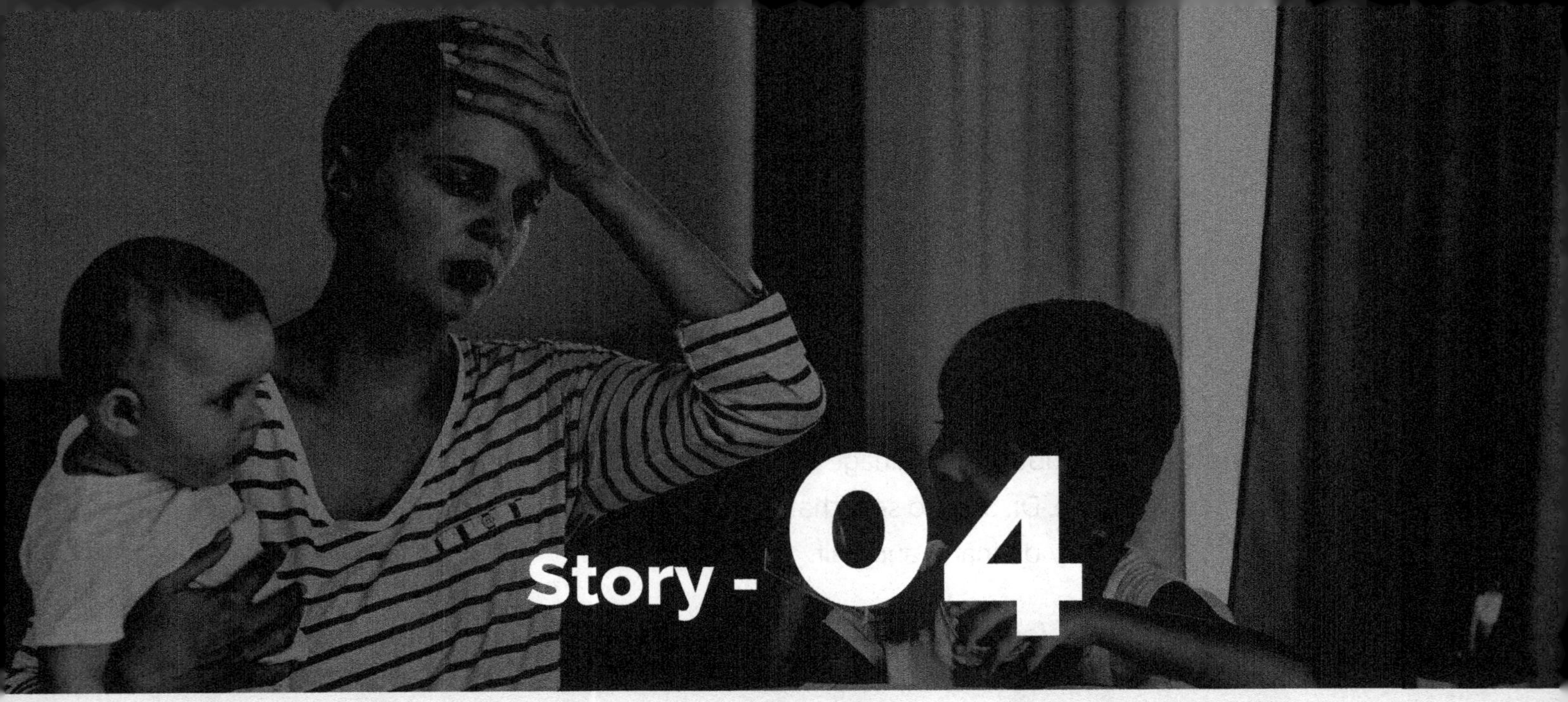

Stubborn Eye Fatigue that Won't Resolve

Deidre spent most of her time reading schoolbooks or doing online homework problems. She was in her second year of college and planned to graduate after three and a half years. That meant she took a few extra classes during the summers, but it was a lot more stressful. This last summer had been brutal between working and schoolwork. As her fall classes approached, she found that her desire to be as dedicated to her classes had waned slightly. She was frustrated by this and vowed to do better. She chalked it up to some slight burnout.

About three weeks into the new semester, the temperature outside dropped, and Deidre wanted to go to a movie rather than schoolwork. She had worked hard for the first three days of the week but needed a night off. She gave herself one more hour of studying, then called her friends and made plans. They picked up some food from the dollar menu and headed to the movie theater.

Once inside, she laughed and joked with her friends. It was good to get out and feel like she was doing something she wanted. She was starting to think it wouldn't be harmful to relax a little on her schoolwork and maybe take fewer classes. Why did she need to push herself so hard to graduate early?

The lights dimmed down, and the movie started. Within twenty minutes, Deidre had a stabbing pain behind her eyes. This lasted for ten minutes, and then it went away. For the next several minutes, she noticed that her eyes were slightly sensitive to the light, and her vision worsened. It got so bad that she had to get up to use the bathroom. When she came back, her vision was mostly better. She wondered if she had just had her first migraine. Her mom had migraines, significantly worse around her menstrual periods.

The movie ended, and Deidre and her friends went their separate ways. The following day, she was back to her usual self. However, over the next few weeks, she discovered her eyes would become fatigued when she was reading or looking at things far away. She went online and found some articles about overtaxed eyes and eye strain. She learned that her eyes might be getting tired due to driving, reading, fatigue, or overusing digital devices.

She bought a pair of blue light glasses from an online store to help with the eye strain. Deidre finished the semester, but her headaches and eye strain were substantially worse during her final exams. She had begun to worry that maybe her vision had changed. She called and set up an appointment with an eye doctor for a visit.

Doctor Becky, the Ophthalmologist, was pleasant. She listened to Deidre's complaints and symptoms and agreed with some of her conclusions.

"Have you ever had an eye exam before?" asked Doctor Becky.

"Maybe years ago," said Deidre. "But I don't remember much."

"It's pretty simple. I will check the pressure in your eye first. We will look at some of your light sensitivity and get a good look at the pupil itself. It means we will need to put some drops in your eye. Then we will do a test to see how your vision is. Does that sound good?"

"Sure."

The exam went flawlessly. But Doctor Becky couldn't find any change in her vision. Everything else was normal as well.

"So?" asked Deidre.

"You have 20/20 vision. There were no problems or other issues that were seen."

"What does that mean?"

"Well...with eye strain, the permanent vision doesn't change. The fatigue causes blurriness, but rest should fix the problem. Maybe if you avoid reading for Christmas break and avoid excessive amounts of time on your phone, you'll see an improvement when you start up classes again. If not, let me know."

Doctor Becky also recommended some eye drops.

Deidre had no issues during the rest of her break. But, when classes started again, the blurriness and headaches started back up again. Deidre called Doctor Becky immediately.

Doctor Becky said, "This is curious. I am a little surprised, but maybe we are looking at this a little wrongly."

"What do you mean?"

"Maybe this doesn't have anything to do with your eyesight. My recommendation is that you get a brain scan. This will help us look at the entire picture."

"If you think so," said Deidre, but she was more worried than ever.

Two weeks later, Deidre went to a local hospital and had a brain scan. It took another week before Doctor Becky called her back into her office. By this point, Deidre felt helpless. Her headaches were worse, and her blurriness was nearly daily, even on weekends. Her grades had slipped, and she was frustrated.

Diedre asked her mom to join her for the visit. Deidre asked, "Did the scans show us anything helpful."

"They did, but it took me some time to talk with a specialist to figure out the best treatment for you."

"Is it something bad?" asked Deidre.

"Not terrible, but something is causing your vision changes, headaches, and more. If left untreated, it could get worse."

"Is it cancer?" asked Deidre. "I've been researching brain cancers and found they can cause symptoms similar to mine."

"No. It's not cancer. There is something that we believe is causing the problems. It isn't eye fatigue though that is one of the primary symptoms, among others."

"What was found?"

"On the brain scan, there is something called an Osteoma. This is not cancer or something inside the brain that is putting pressure on your brain. You aren't at risk for seizures or other complications. The Osteoma is a benign head tumor that is like extra growth on your skull."

"Ouch. That sounds painful," replied Deidre. "But a tumor doesn't sound like a good thing."

"Well...it depends on the meaning behind the tumor. In this case, it is not cancerous, and sometimes it doesn't even need treatment."

"I can't live like this," said Deidra. "I feel miserable all the time."

"I know. That is why I called someone and talked to him about the possible treatments. He also looked at the scan. He recommends that we do surgery to remove the piece of bone causing the problems. Its location is probably causing inflammation and other issues, especially when you are reading a lot. He worries that without treatment, your symptoms will get worse."

"What's the treatment?"

"Surgery. It is called the Expanded Endonasal Approach or EEA. This is a minimally invasive surgical technique where they go through your nose and remove the tumor. They kind of half to go through your sinus cavity. It sounds worse than it is. You will stay overnight in the hospital for one day, and you should be able to go home the next day."

"If you say so."

"Once you're on the other side of this, you'll be thrilled you had the surgery."

"Let's do it."

A few weeks later, during spring break, Deidra was checked into the hospital for surgery. Like before, she was worried, but Doctor Becky's encouragement and meeting with the surgeon alleviated much of her stress. The surgery went perfectly, and she went home and rested the remainder of her time away from school.

Additionally, she was able to resume her studies without much of a delay. Her symptoms resolved, and she became excited about her studies again. Her worse remaining symptom was an occasional nosebleed. She still graduated early.

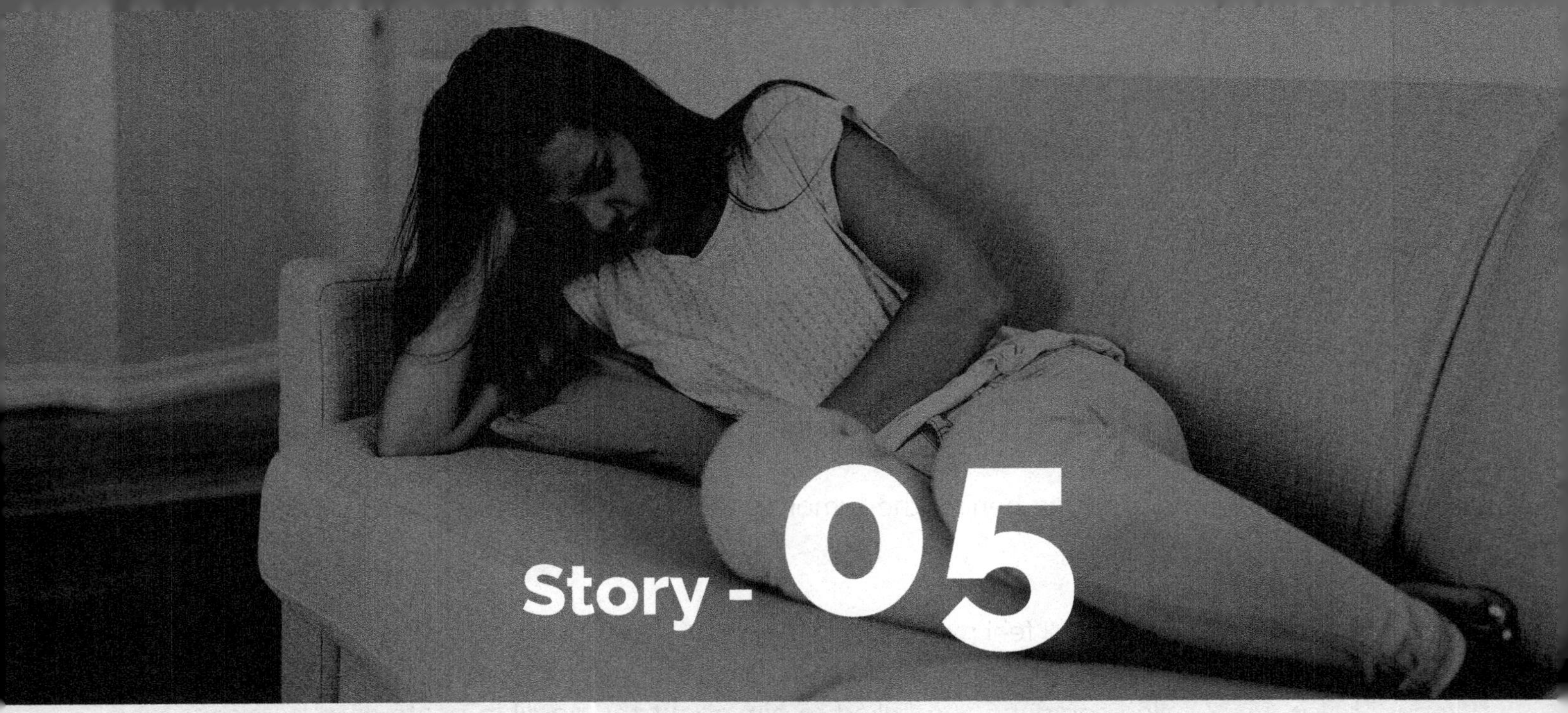

Story - 05

Struggles with an Abdominal Hernia

Caroline was active at church, her part-time job, with her husband and three kids, and in her neighborhood. She loved to work out with Zumba and run. When she turned forty-five, she started lifting weights once or twice a week to keep active and gain muscle. She was worried about the osteoporosis that her mother suffered from. She joined an excellent group online and started to improve her eating. She found incredible recipes and counted her macros.

For the first six months, she saw minimal improvements. She felt significantly better; drinking water made her mind clearer, and her stomach was less bloated. Occasionally she would have some sharp pains in her stomach, and it would take a few days for her to have a bowel movement. She added fiber to her diet and as a gummy, which improved things.

Ten months after starting this new program, she was lifting at her gym with some of her friends one day. While doing some squats while holding a kettlebell, she felt some tightness in her stomach. She didn't think much of it and finished her set. She rested and drank some water as the other girls took their turns. When it was her turn again, she bent down for the first squat, but it was clear that she couldn't continue.

"You've stained your abdomen," said one of her close friends.

It sounded right, and honestly, Caroline could not do any more lifting the rest of the day. The next day, the pain was slightly worse, but she could move around. She avoided any exercise for the next few days. Over the following two weeks, the pain slowly improved. It took her another two weeks before she started lifting again. She did stretches and running, and her pain was minimal.

Two months later, she was back to her usual self, but one day she noticed a small lump in her belly button area. She didn't think she had seen it before but couldn't be sure. When she pushed on it, it was really tender. She called her doctor and set up an appointment.

Before the visit, she thought she knew what might be going on. She had several other people tell her their opinions. When Doctor McDaniel came in and performed an exam. She was unsurprised when he said, "I think you have an abdominal hernia, more specifically called an umbilical hernia. We can order an ultrasound to confirm."

"Should I be worried?" asked Caroline.

"I wouldn't be. It's a little tender right now. That could go away."

"Do I need surgery?"

"Maybe. Not everyone does. We will see how things go in the next few months."

"Should I be worried?"

"Normally, no. Most of these types of hernias don't cause huge problems. But you need to let us know if something changes. If you get more pain, or it gets bigger, or you notice any redness."

"I think I can do that."

The next six months were relatively normal. There wasn't a change in the size of the hernia or increased pain. That changed one night during a vacation when she had been outside most of the day. Rick, her husband, and she had escaped to the beach for a few days. She hadn't felt any pain during the day, but she thought she might have overdone something. She wasn't too worried but kept an eye on her pain level. The pain didn't improve at all, and the pain worsened considerably over the next three days. To make matters worse, the hernia doubled in size.

When Caroline returned from her vacation, she called Dr. McDaniel, and he scheduled another ultrasound.

The nurse for Dr. McDaniel called her to come for an appointment to tell her the news. Again, she was unsurprised when she heard Dr. Daniel say, "The hernia is bigger than before. I think it might be best if we get a surgical consult to see if you should get surgery."

"Okay."

"I'll refer you to Dr. Montgomery. She is the best."

Caroline met with Dr. Montgomery three weeks later, and it was determined that surgery was required. The surgical date was put on the calendar for another three weeks from that day. Dr. Montgomery explained the procedure and the recovery time. It wasn't horrible, and she was hopeful that she would be back exercising by the first part of the summer. Dr. Montgomery also did a great job answering all of her questions and decreasing her anxiety about the procedure.

Three weeks later, the surgery date arrived. Caroline's husband drove her to the hospital, and they checked in. Dr. Montgomery came and talked to her for a few minutes after they had checked in and were given a bed. She confirmed that she was ready, hadn't eaten, and still wanted to proceed with the surgery.

She was told the surgery would require an hour, maybe a little more. She would remain in recovery for a few hours and then go home. She would be restricted in how much she could pick up for the first few weeks. She wouldn't be able to do strenuous activity until four to six weeks after the procedure.

"Let's roll," said Caroline.

After surgery, when Caroline awoke, she found herself in recovery. Her husband was close by talking with Dr. Montgomery. She barely remembered coming out of surgery but had fallen back to sleep quickly. Now, her mind felt clearer. She asked, "How did it go?"

Dr. Montgomery turned and said, "I was just telling your husband, Rick, that things were more difficult than anticipated."

"What does that mean?"

"The surgery took over two hours. We had planned on doing everything arthroscopically, but when we got inside, it looked like there was some additional tissue involved. Despite our initial attempts, we were forced to open up the abdomen with a bigger incision to repair the hernia."

"Were you successful?"

"Yes," replied Dr. Montgomery, but she glanced at Rick. "There was a lot of bleeding, more than usual, and the added tissue made things a little more difficult. The recovery time we talked about before will be a little longer. You have a larger incision site than we planned."

"How large are we talking?" asked Caroline.

"About five inches."

"Will it leave a scar?"

"Yes, it will. I'm sorry."

"It's fine."

Rick added, "I'm sure everything will look great."

"One last thing," noted Dr. Montgomery. "We sent some of the extra tissue to a pathologist to take a look. I'm sure it is nothing, but I've never seen that much extra tissue in a hernia before. That will take about a week to get back."

Caroline remained in recovery for the next few hours. Her pain became surprisingly strong before she left, but she was able to have a bowel movement that was a little runny. It took some effort to get into the wheelchair as she was not able to walk on her own.

The next few weeks were brutal. The healing process was slow and cumbersome. It became frustrating for Caroline that she was not able to do things on her own. The incision site was healing okay, but it was painful every time she laughed, moved, or went to the bathroom. She was surprised that the bloating got worse, but she assumed that it was from the pain medications.

Dr. McDaniel's office called a few times to check up on Caroline. Two weeks after surgery, Dr. McDaniel called and asked for Caroline and Rick to come to his office for a check-up. The call was early in the morning and they arrived at the office around eleven a.m.

They were brought back to an exam room almost immediately, and soon Dr. McDaniel and Dr. Montgomery stepped into the room. Caroline was surprised to see both at the same time.

Dr. Montgomery asked, "How is the healing process?"

Caroline explained what she was able and not able to do. She described the pain in her stomach, abdomen, and sometimes when she went to the bathroom. Soon, Dr. Montgomery performed an exam on the incision site and pushed her stomach in different places.

Once finished, Dr. McDaniel asked, "How is your energy level? How are you eating? How are your bowel movements?"

Caroline answered each.

Once she was finished, Dr. Montgomery said, "We got the results back from the tissue biopsy."

"Is that why both of her doctors are here?" asked Rick.

"Yes," said Dr. Montgomery. "Unfortunately. There is no better way to say this than, to be honest. The findings show an aggressive form of cancer. We've never seen it before in a hernia, and it is important to understand that the hernia certainly didn't cause this. In fact, without the hernia, by the time it was discovered, it would be far too late."

The results blindsided Caroline. Never in her life had she expected this diagnosis. They talked a lot about her subtle symptoms of feeling fatigued, sharp pains, bloating, bowel movement changes, and more.

"What's the plan?" asked Rick. "How do we make her better?"

"The chances that she'll recover completely are very low. We can try some chemotherapy, and that could shrink the cancer. Maybe another surgery, but chances are that this will get the best of her in the end."

"So, the surgery made her worse?" demanded Rick.

"No. She would not have lived for another three months had she not had the surgery. Now, we can push back her life expectance for maybe two years."

Caroline went with treatment, and for the most part, she did exceptionally well. She had some poor days and some good days, but she lived two years, six months past the date of diagnosis, and tried to enjoy every moment.

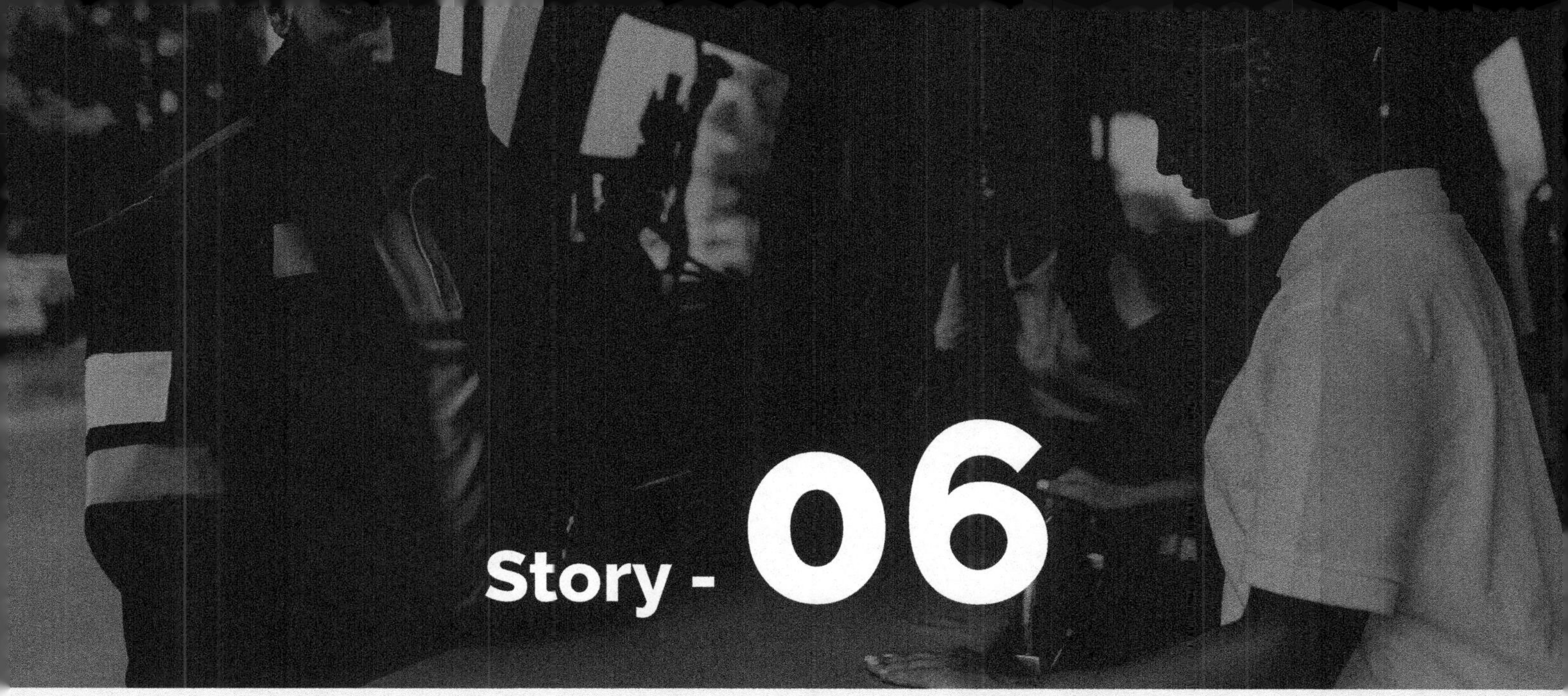

Story - 06

The Frat Party Challenge

The ambulance arrived at the hospital's front door, and an unconscious, barely breathing young man was transported out of the back and into the hospital. Shortly after that, a car with two young men arrived, and they insisted that they were friends and roommates with the person who was brought in—just a few minutes earlier. They demanded to know what was wrong with their roommate.

The two roommates were taken to a side room to get more information about the unconscious boy. I was called to the ER room to help. When I arrived, the patient was in a full seizure. His entire body was shaking. I was told that his name was Derek Conners.

The doctor shouted, "We need to give Narcan."

Standing next to Dr. Abram, Nurse Stevens opened a drawer and pulled out the Narcan. It was a nasal spray and was given inside the nose. After two minutes, there was no change.

Dr. Abram said, "Give another dose of Narcan, and we need 2mg of Ativan. Get some oxygen and start an IV."

I hurried off to gather the medication and the necessary supplies. I rushed back in just as Nurse Fayda finished the set-up for the IV. She was excellent in these traumatic events, with the patient flopping or moving. The boy was tall and muscular but not overweight. The flip was switched, and the fluids went in as quickly as possible.

I said, "Ativan is here."

"Give now."

I moved in as other staff members held down the boy. I administered the medication without any problems. Fluids were started, and blood was taken. The patient's seizures stopped for a few minutes but started back up again. It took more fluids and some additional medications to control the seizures. Despite everything we were trying, the patient would not wake up, even after the attacks stopped.

It did not take long before Dr. Abrams became concerned with how the patient was presenting and the inability to get him to respond that he was placed in a drug-induced coma. The patient was stable, breathing, and the heart rate was slightly elevated. There were some slight abnormal changes on EKG. We needed more information.

I accompanied Dr. Abrams into the room with the two roommates. Dr. Abrams asked, "Can you tell me what happened? Any drug use, overdose, or medications?"

Jack, one of the roommates, said, "Jeff and I have been at classes most of the day. Derek had the day off, and he was chilling at the apartment. He was tired when we arrived after class. We played some video games, and everything seemed fine. He didn't feel like eating dinner and just lay on the couch. The next thing we knew, he started jerking weirdly, and we couldn't get him to wake up."

Jeff added, "I splashed some water on his face and pushed him, but nothing. That was when we called for an ambulance."

"Any drug use?" I asked again.

"A little marijuana but not today."

"What about prescription pills for pain, anxiety, or anything else?"

Jack glanced at Jeff, and the two shrugged. Jeff answered, "Derek doesn't use drugs, as far as I know."

The door opened, and Nurse Fayda asked for Dr. Abrams and me to step from the room. We did, and she said, "We got some of the preliminary labs back. Derek Clayton has a critically high sodium level."

"How high?"

"Higher than I've seen in a long time."

"Are we giving him NS (Normal Saline)?"

"Yes," I answered, and the three of us hurried back to Derek's room. He was still unconscious, and Nurse Stevens was there getting a set of vitals.

Dr. Abrams said, "Let's change that to D5 (Dextrose 5%). We need to stop the NS because it has sodium in it, making the problem worse. We need to place a Foley catheter."

Nurse Stevens asked, "What's going on?"

I explained the results of the blood test.

"Why is his sodium so high?"

"That's the question," I replied. I helped Nurse Stevens place the Foley catheter while Nurse Fayda changed the NS for D5.

"He doesn't seem dehydrated," said Dr. Abrams. "His roommates didn't say anything about him having significant diarrhea. We need to get an abdominal CT."

The next few hours were spent doing test after test. We checked kidney function, heart risks, liver problems, and much more. The blood work, especially the sodium, started to improve after three hours or more of intense fluids.

When the CT of the abdomen came back, it was also normal. Dr. Abrams and I returned to speak with Jack and Jeff.

When we stepped into the room, Jeff asked, "How is Derek doing?"

"He seems to be doing a little better."

"Can we talk with him?"

"He is in a medicated coma for now. He started having some seizures, and we don't know why. His blood work showed that his sodium level was extremely high. Everything else has been normal. Would you happen to know why his sodium level is so high?"

"Sodium means salt, right?" asked Jack.

"Exactly," replied Dr. Abrams.

Jack shook his head. "Derek doesn't really put a lot of salt on his food. We haven't been out to eat. I have no idea why he has some much salt in his blood."

I asked, "What about excessive drinking or diarrhea."

"Water or alcohol?"

"Either."

"Derek works out and drinks a lot of water. We went to a party last night, but I don't think he drank at all," said Jeff.

I was about to leave the room when Dr. Abrams asked, "Tell me about the last few days."

"We all had classes the last three days. Tomorrow is Friday, and we have some plans," said Jeff. "Monday, we hung out with some friends and watched football. We bought some wings. Tuesday was a frat party, and we went and hung out there most of the night. Jack, me, and Derek started playing some games. It was fun."

"What kind of games?"

"Challenges and ticktock videos. We would get videoed doing weird and crazy things."

"Like what?" I asked.

Jack added, "We weren't the only ones. Several people were doing it. It was like a contest between two groups."

"What kind of challenges?"

Jeff laughed, "I had to eat a bunch of hot dogs."

"I tried drinking a gallon of milk," added Jack.

"Did Derek try anything?"

"I think so," Jeff said. "But I'm not sure what it was."

"I think he had to drink something after I did. I don't know what happened because I started puking up the milk."

"We can check out phones," said Jeff. "I am sure that someone videoed it."

Ten minutes later, Jeff found the video and showed it to Dr. Abram and me. A group of kids in a house stood around a healthy-appearing Derek. They were chanting, "Drink. Drink! Drink!"

A dark liquid was poured from a large container. Derek began drinking glass after glass. His face contorted as he swallowed his third glass. My stomach became ill just watching it."

"That would do it," said Dr. Abram. "It appears that Derek was challenged to drink as much Soy sauce as possible. That is filled with a ton of salt."

Derek stayed in an induced coma for four days. He was pumped with D5 to clear out the sodium, which took almost 24 hours. He was taken out of the coma, and it took several hours for him to fully wake. He remembered nothing of what had happened to him and why he was in the hospital. Dr. Abrams explained that his challenge of drinking Soy sauce had induced seizures, some brain swelling, and an inability for us to wake him up. He was shocked that drinking Soy sauce could have caused him to go into a coma.

"I'm not sure I'll ever touch that stuff again," he said as he was discharged a few days later with no lasting problems.

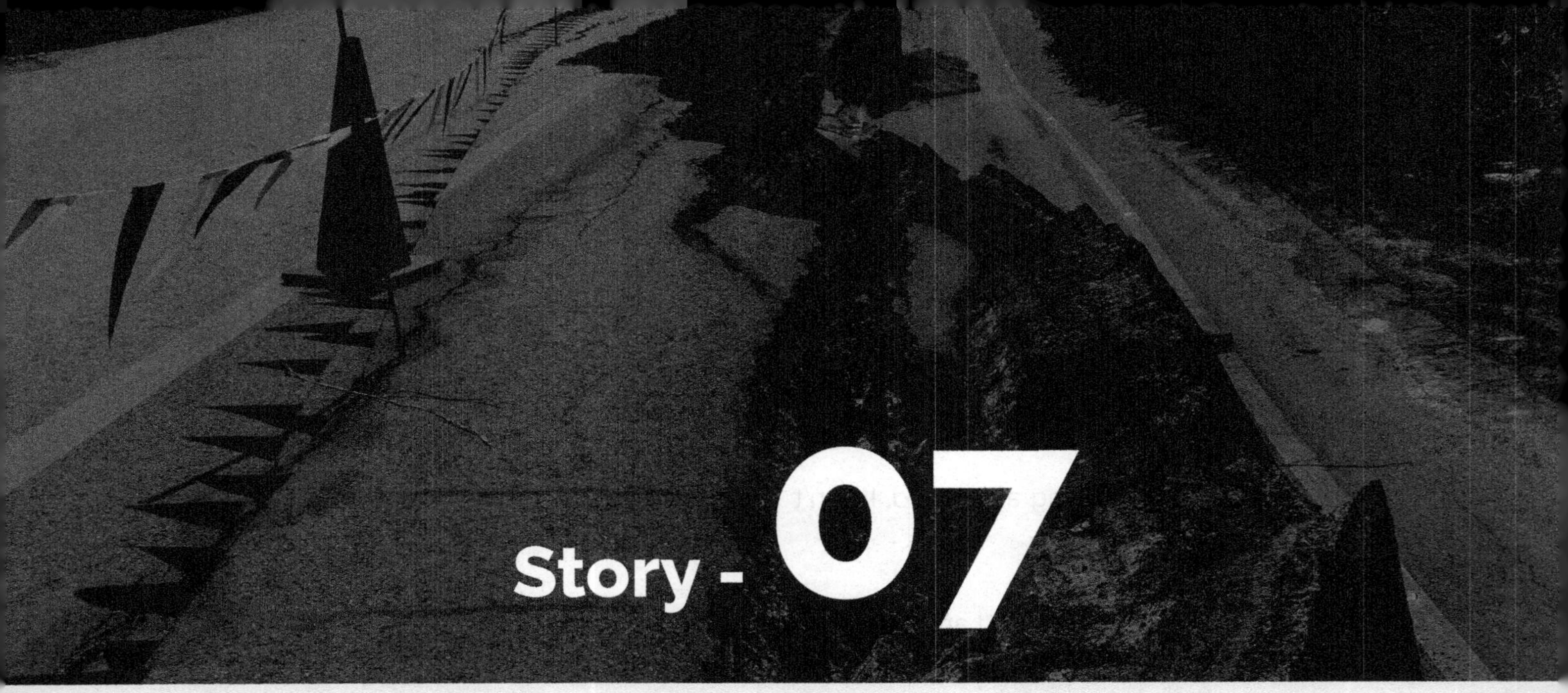

Story - 07

An Early Spring Canyon Crash

911 operator, "Hello. This is dispatch. Are you calling to report an emergency?"

A male voice responded, clearly out of breath, "Yes. My girlfriend and I were in an accident up Stinger Canyon. There was some debris on the road, and it was icy. I crashed. I think the car flipped a few times. I was able to pull myself free. She is still stuck. She is in bad shape. Send an ambulance."

"Are you injured, sir?"

"I don't know." There was a pause. "Maybe. My arm isn't moving right, and it throbs."

"We will send some help."

"Hurry. I think she is stuck. It's freezing out here."

"Do you remember where you crashed?"

"Not really. It was like the third bend in the road."

"We've contacted the ambulance and Search and Rescue, and they're on their way. Can you remember anything around you?"

"Not really," the male replied. "But the car landed upside down in the water. Please hurry."

The line went dead.

The debris, a dead deer, was still on the road when the ambulance arrived. There were tire marks, and it was apparent where the car had left the road. The canyon was closed in both directions, and Search and Rescue began unpacking their gear. It took less than ten minutes for a five-person team to get dressed, grab their equipment, and descend to the ravine. There was snowy and icy, but the worst part was the temperature. It took another three or four minutes to find the car.

The water wasn't deep, and they could hear someone crying.

"Help me!" the girl screamed.

"We're here," replied one of the rescuers.

"I'm stuck," she added. "I'm so cold."

"What's your name?"

"Tammy," she said. "Have you seen my fiancé?"

"We haven't. But I think he was the one who called in the accident. We'll start looking for him once we get you secured."

"I can't get the seatbelt off. There is a lot of blood in my eyes."

"My name is Derek. I'm going to take a look at you from the passenger's seat." Derek hurried forward. He found the side door open. From this angle, it was clear that Tammy had more risks from the stream than her boyfriend did. If it had been later in the spring, the water would have been higher, and Tammy likely would have drowned upside down in her car. The vehicle was also tilted slightly so that opening the driver's door would be impossible without lifting up the car. That was not an option in this canyon.

As he crawled into the car, he noticed some of Tammy's injuries. She was severely injured, with possible broken bones and cuts, and she was having trouble catching her breath, and there was a gash on her head. Derek asked, "How's your breathing?"

"It's hard for me to take a deep breath. Is that bad?"

"It might be the fact that you're upside down. But you could have injured your lungs or your ribs. You've had quite the accident."

Tammy began to cry at these words as if the truth of the dire situation washed her misbeliefs away. She knew she was in bad shape.

"You're going to be fine," said Derek hastily. "Don't panic. That won't help. We can get you out. I need to cut you from your seatbelt and pull you out this side."

"Where is my fiancé?" she asked again.

"He's fine. He called 911 to report the accident."

"I want to see him," Tammy insisted.

"Once you are safe from this accident. For now, you need to worry about yourself."

"Is there something wrong with me?"

"Nothing that we can't fix," answered Derek.

The next twenty minutes were spent on getting Tammy from the vehicle. Her extraction was done in phases. First, the safety harness was removed, and Derek checked her neck and back. She was stable, and upon first glance, it didn't appear she had severely injured her neck or back.

Once she was released from the belt, it took a few moments to lift her clear of the console and where her feet were positioned, close to the peddles. The paramedics had brought down a gurney, and when Tammy was removed from the car, she was immediately placed on a backboard and stabilized onto the gurney. This was a typical procedure and precautionary. It took four people to carry her from the scene of the accident.

The incident commander asked Derek, "How is she?"

"Hurt and injured. I think she might have an injury to her head, possibly broken bones, but she is talking and makes sense...most of the time."

"Have we found her fiancé?" asked the incident commander.

"Not as far as I've heard. We will keep looking.

Tammy was carried up the hill and over to the ambulance. She was quickly placed inside. An IV was initiated as the ambulance drove back into town. It would take thirty minutes to get to the hospital. Once the ambulance arrived, they had staff waiting. Tammy had taken a turn for the worse and was having trouble breathing on her own. Oxygen was placed.

Inside the hospital, it became clear that one of her lungs had been damaged. She had fluid on her lungs and couldn't wholly expand when she exhaled and inhaled.

She required a chest tube to be inserted. This was necessary on the left side. Doctor Joseph and Nurse Vance performed the procedure. The plastic tube was inserted into the left lung. Blood had pooled in the lower part of the lung and some of the chest wall.

The X-ray revealed that she had four broken ribs, one of which had punctured the lung. The chest tube alone would not be adequate treatment. She would need surgery to repair the broken rib. To make matters worse, Tammy was still worsening when it came to her responsiveness. It wasn't because of the lack of oxygen, but she had a skull fracture and increased pressure on the brain.

Both injuries were potentially life-threatening. Tammy was brought to surgery, and four hours later, she came out of surgery with a greater chance of survival.

The following day she woke up. The doctor, her parents, and her sister were there.

Doctor Joseph asked, "Tammy. How are you feeling?"

"I don't know. I'm tired, and I can't move. What's wrong with me?"

Both of her parents started to cry.

Doctor Joseph came closer and started examining her. The bandage on her head was well-placed. Her ribs were bandaged, and she still had a chest tube. He looked at her eyes, and they responded well to light. She had some facial bruising and a broken arm. Doctor Joseph asked, "What do you remember from the accident?"

She tried to shake her head back and forth. When she realized she couldn't move, she asked, "What's wrong with me?"

"What do you remember?" he encouraged.

It appeared as if Tammy were thinking. She finally answered, "A crash. Up the canyon. I was stuck."

Doctor Joseph nodded. "You broke some ribs, and you had a head injury. When you arrived at the hospital, you were hurt, and we had to do surgery on your lungs and your head."

Tammy's facial features changed, and her voice was faint when she asked, "Where is my fiancé?"

"He escaped the car crash and called 911 for help."

"He got out of the car?" Tammy asked, clearly confused.

"He did."

"Can I see him?"

"Well," Doctor Joseph sat on a chair next to her bed. "It took them longer to find him. He was out in the elements for a few hours. He had been wet. He had an episode of hypothermia."

"What does that mean?"

"He was less injured by the car accident but more susceptible to sickness from the hypothermia."

"Where is he?"

"He is in a drug-induced coma. But he is responding well to treatment. We are hopeful he will be awake in a few days."

"So...he's okay."

"We don't know for sure, but we will keep you updated."

Tammy's recovery took weeks. Her fiancé's recovery took longer. Both were injured but differently, and they would never be the same. The fiancé had some problems with frostbite, a dislocated shoulder, and a broken arm. They couldn't do surgery for two weeks after the accident because of the hypothermia. Tammy's brain injury was a TBI, and she suffered from short-term memory loss. With work, she improved this over the next few years, but it never completely went away.

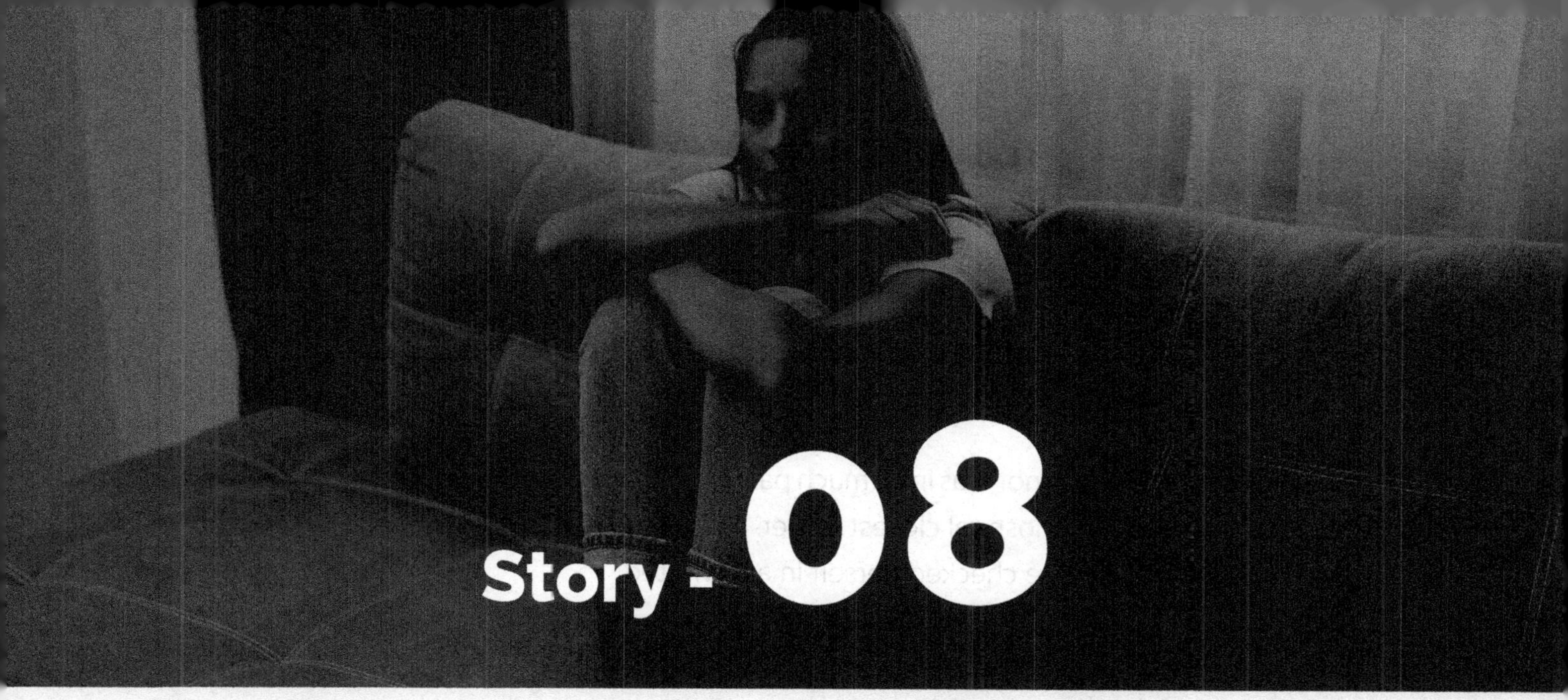

Feeling too Embarrassed to Tell Someone About the Pain

Eleanor Blanchard went to her family doctor for a routine checkup. She needed some refills of medications and blood work and wanted to discuss getting her IUD removed. She and her husband had been tossing around the idea of getting pregnant, and she wanted to be ready.

During the visit, she spoke about everything that she needed to talk about, except the most painful problem that she was having. She had a pap smear and an IUD removal, and when she squirmed in pain at each and every movement, she blamed her pain on the fact that she was nervous about getting the IUD removed. It was far from the truth.

She got a prescription for oral birth control until she and her husband were ready. Her other medications were filled, and she thanked the doctor and left. At the door, she stopped and wondered if she should go back inside and tell the truth about her problems.

A week later, she sat back and prepared for the Botox on her chin, forehead, and lip lines. She had been getting Botox for three years and looked forward to it each time. The aesthetician that did the procedure was professional and polite, unlike the one that had been there a year before. That girl had been shady, or at least that was what Eleanor believed today after everything that had happened.

Eleanor wondered what the pretty girl working on her face would think if she knew the entire truth. She wanted to tell her all the agony Eleanor was feeling. Maybe it would make her feel better, maybe it wouldn't. She was too humiliated. She left the appointment feeling both rejuvenated and dejected. She should have told someone.

Another month passed, and Eleanor was in so much pain that she had no choice but to go to the emergency room. Instead of driving to the hospital closest to her, she drove another two hours to a sister hospital on the opposite side of the city. She checked herself in and waited.

A few hours later, she was brought back to a room and waited for the nurse to come to check on her.

Nurse Fillmore arrived, "Hello, Eleanor Blanchard. What seems to be the matter?"

"It's my stomach," said Eleanor calmly. "I had an IUD removed a few weeks ago, and my stomach and kidneys have been on fire over the last few weeks. I thought it would go away, but it hasn't."

"What kind of IUD did you have?"

"Mirena."

"Why did you have it placed initially and why was it removed?"

"My husband and I weren't ready for children. It was used for birth control. Lately, we've been thinking about increasing the size of our family."

"Any chance you have endometriosis or a similar problem?"

Eleanor shook her head.

"Have you been using other protection? Could you be pregnant?"

"I'm on the second month of my oral contraceptives. I haven't missed a day. My pain is really in my kidneys."

"I will go tell the doctor, and he'll stop by in a few minutes."

"Thank you."

Doctor York arrived and asked similar questions. Eleanor answered them the same as she had done before. Doctor York was young, attractive, and a man. Eleanor wished she had been assigned a female doctor. The exam was done, and Eleanor slightly exaggerated her stomach symptoms, especially on her right kidney. She was in pain; she just wasn't being completely honest about its location. She wanted to check herself out of the hospital and never come back.

Doctor York said, "Let's do an ultrasound on her pelvis and both kidneys. Let's get a urine sample and some blood work. Let's see if we're dealing with a kidney stone or an infection."

"Sounds great," said Eleanor.

Twenty minutes later, Nurse Fillmore returned and drew the blood. Eleanor was allowed to go into the bathroom and provide a urine sample. She walked gingerly to the bathroom and back again, and her movements were filled with intense pain. She wasn't faking that at all.

Another thirty minutes passed before the Ultrasound tech came in. Eleanor lifted her shirt, exposing her stomach. The tech started with the central lower part of her stomach. The first ultrasound took the longest, and extreme discomfort was felt as she pushed the probe into her stomach.

The tech asked, "Does that hurt?"

Eleanor nodded. But the pain wasn't in her stomach, but she refused to voice that fact.

The kidneys were checked next. Thankfully, she felt less pain during these tests. As the tech was leaving, she said, "Hope you fill better."

Eleanor smiled.

An hour later, Eleanor was starting to feel nervous about her complicity in the tests that were run. She knew they would all come back normal, and she was too afraid to explain the real problem. She stood and started getting dressed. There was a knock at the door.

"Just a minute," said Eleanor, and she tore off her jeans, causing even more pain, and jumped back into bed. Her eyes filled with tears due to the pain. Taking a few deep breaths, she tried settling her nerves. Finally, she said, "Come in."

Doctor York, Nurse Fillmore, and two other people in white coats entered the room. They were also male, young, and wide-eyed.

"Hello, Mrs. Blanchard. I've asked Doctors Calder and Avery to accompany me."

"Okay," said Eleanor. "Is there something wrong?"

"Not really. Both are students, and you're a slightly unusual case."

"Unusual?" replied Eleanor.

"You're reporting some pain in the pelvic area and the kidneys. The tech noticed how much pain you were in during the ultrasound."

"I was just uncomfortable." She glanced around the room. "Was there a problem?"

"The ultrasounds of your bladder, ovaries, and kidneys were completely normal. The urine doesn't show any infection. You have no kidney stones, and it doesn't appear you have a kidney infection."

"That's a relief."

"But," said Doctor York. "Your blood work showed that you likely have a serious infection. Your white count is really high."

"What does white count mean?"

"It is one of the blood tests we do, and in this case, it shows a possible infection. It isn't just a little high, but extremely high. We're just a little confused that we might be missing something. Do you have any problems with diarrhea, sweats, hot or cold flashes, breathing issues, or anything else? Have you ever had your gallbladder removed?"

"No..." Eleanor said hesitantly. She felt all the eyes of the room were on her, and she suddenly burst into tears.

Nurse Fillmore came and sat on the edge of the bed. She tried consoling Eleanor but was shocked at the response.

Eleanor cried for another few minutes. Once she had recovered, she muttered, "I've made the biggest mistake of my life."

"Mistake," said Doctor York. "What do you mean?"

"I get Botox every three or four weeks."

"I don't think Botox caused whatever is happening," said Nurse Filmore kindly.

"I know. But I was talking with the girl helping me with my Botox one day. I told her that I wanted butt injections to give me a lift. I had looked into it before, but it was so expensive. She said she knew someone who could help, and the cost would be way less."

"Go on," said Doctor York.

"She introduced me to a friend of a friend. He said that he had cutting-edge technology and that monthly injections would provide all that I would need."

"How long ago did this start?"

"One year."

Nurse Fillmore asked, "How much pain are you in?"

"Significant," said Eleanor. "The injections started out fine. I was told that they would be silicone. The first three were perfect, and I loved how they looked, but after a few more months, they started to shrink a little. I called them back and scheduled some more injections."

Doctor York asked, "What did they say when you called them back?"

"That silicone injections can settle a little, like the foundation of a house. But on the next few sets of injections, my body reacted badly, and I started having some redness, and pain, and it wasn't as smooth as it was before."

"How long ago was that?" asked Nurse Fillmore

"Six months."

"You've been in pain for six months."

"The last three have been the worst."

"Can we take a look?" asked Doctor York.

"I'm so embarrassed with how it looks."

Nurse Fillmore helped Eleanor stand. "Don't worry about a thing, hun."

The room became dead quiet as Eleanor showed her backside. She had bruising, redness, and the skin was warm to the touch. The left side was worse than the right, but both sides had significant problems.

"Well," said Doctor York. "I think we know why your blood work was so abnormal."

"Do you think an antibiotic will help?" asked Eleanor.

"Honestly. You're going to need a lot more than an antibiotic. Those implants, or whatever was placed into your buttocks, will need to be removed. You're going to need surgery and be admitted to the hospital."

"My husband is going to kill me. He loved the idea initially of the butt lift, but he told me to stop going back. I wished I'd listened."

The surgery took eight hours. In addition to the silicone implant removal, some of the dead tissue was also removed. There was infection and hardening of some of the tissue. The process was not pretty. The wounds were kept open for a few days, and a wound vac was used to clean out most of the infection. Eleanor was on IV antibiotics for three weeks.

Five days after the initial surgery, Eleanor had a second one to clean out more dead tissue. There had been some healing, and the wound was closed at that point. Two weeks later, she was discharged home with strict instructions to avoid lifting and moving too much.

It took Eleanor months to heal from the ordeal of infection, surgery, and removal of the implants. She lost a lot of blood, and the surgery to fix things was done as best as they could, but the scars would remain forever. However, she was lucky to have survived. She later learned that other women had done similar things and had a far less favorable outcome. She learned that feeling embarrassed was far better than feeling that sick.

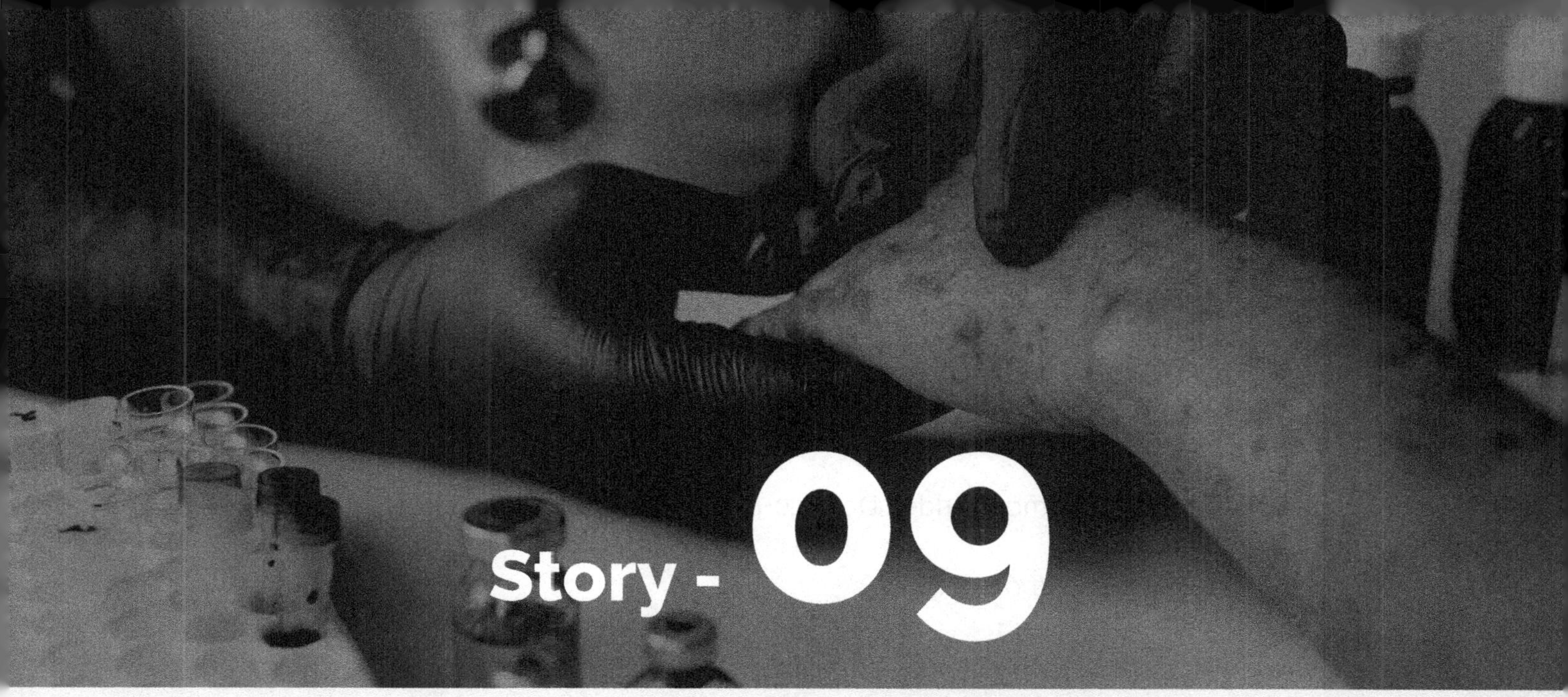

Story - 09

Severe Scratches of the Skin

The prison administration worked for many months to facilitate the transfer of one of their inmates to a prison closer to where his family lives. This doesn't always work out, but our inmate had just received the news that he had cancer and his parents' health was failing. The parole board approved the paperwork, and he was sent on a bus with two officers, and it took three days to arrive without incident.

Whenever this type of transfer happens, the jail will often receive a new inmate from the same facility. Around the same time our inmate was placed on the bus, Desri Stevens was being loaded into a van for the journey to our state. She arrived with a spit hood and cuffs around her waist that connected with her hands and leg irons. The van ride for the three officers was anything but pleasant. She was unruly and difficult, and finding a hotel to accommodate all three officers was challenging. It wouldn't take long for the prison to regret the exchange, at least at first.

I was the nurse that was present when she arrived. We needed to do an intake screening in order to get her medical and mental health background. We also would get a list of medications and do an assessment. If there were any serious problems, we would refer them to the provider to address them.

Desri shuffled into the exam room, and her spit hood was removed. She was angry and tired and did not like the fact that she had been transferred to our state. She made that clear as quickly and as often as possible.

The first thing I noticed was the large gashes on her forehead that had since healed and were now scars. Additionally, she had newer scratch marks on her face, chest, and legs. I began to worry that she had been hurting herself.

I asked, "What are these scratches from?"

"Coming here wasn't exactly a smooth ride," Desri countered. "It's not like I went to Disneyland."

"Were you trying to hurt yourself on purpose?"

"Why would you go thinking that?"

"Some of these scratches are new, and some are older."

"No kidding. Why don't you go kiss my ass."

The remainder of the intake was done in a similar fashion. Each question was repeated back to me, and there was attitude, contempt, and sarcasm. The assessment went as well as possible. The cuffs could not be removed because of her behavior. She threatened to spit on me twice.

Once finished, Desri was placed on suicide watch, and that's when her language skills became apparent. She swore, threatened, and hit the cell wall as if she were picturing my face and trying to destroy it. Her strength and strong word language were impressive.

Mental health came quickly to her cell, and several questions were asked. I was required to stay close, but I remained out of sight. Desri had no idea why she was placed on suicide watch. The social worker tried to get a clearer picture of why she had scratches on her body. Desri was only willing to share a little information, and she never wanted to see that "Stupid nurse again."

It wasn't like I could leave until we were finished. I told Desri that the sooner we were finished, the better for her. Finally, Desri told us that she had depression and some panic attacks. Additionally, she had a medication for high blood pressure and was borderline diabetic. I explained that we might need to do blood work or blood sugar checks. I would consult with the doctor and see if he had any orders.

The next day I had several other intakes from people coming back to the prison or being sent here for the first time. These individuals were not coming from a different state but were brought from local county jails. Once I finished, I went back to check on Desri and some of the other inmates in the section where

I was working. The social worker had stopped by again, and Desir had already been seen by the medical provider. All of her medications had been reordered.

Her mood had drastically changed, and it was staggering. She had showered and gotten some sleep and greeted me kindly. This abrupt change was surprising. She had empty Styrofoam trays and had been drinking. She waved me over and looked ten years younger.

"Thank you, Nurse Campbell, for all you've done for me."

"No problem Desri. You look like you're doing well."

"I slept great last night. I talked with the social worker this morning. She thinks I'm doing good."

"That is so good to hear," I said.

She thanked me for helping her yesterday, and she hoped to be taken off of suicide watch the next day. Her scratch marks were less noticeable, and she looked healthy.

The following day was my last day on the shift for the week. I went through the same process of getting through my intakes. I headed out to see the same people as the day before. When I arrived at Desri's cell, I was confounded that she had transformed back into the person I'd seen the first day. She had new scratches, was angry, and slammed her fist into the wall when she saw me.

Scratch marks covered her face, both arms, and her neck. Some of them were actively bleeding through the gauze placed during the night. Her voice was low and raspy, and she had aged back the ten years from the previous day or more. The charting from the middle of the night reported self-harm, anger issues, and ripping off the first two attempts to clean and dress the wounds.

Looking closer at the charting, the nurse from the night shift noted that sometime around four in the morning, she had flipped out and said that there were bugs all around the room, crawling on her and trying to burrow into her skin. She had freaked out and started pounding on the door, and when the officers arrived, they found several self-injuries. It took several minutes to subdue her, and they even had to give her a shot to calm her down. The officers or nurses saw no bugs or other things inside the cell.

I called down to and control room, and two officers were sent to her cell to help. She cuffed up without incident, but she was angry at me.

"We're going to take you to medical and clean up those wounds."

"Why? The bugs will come back out of my skin when you aren't looking."

"We can try to help you with that."

"No, you can't."

Desri was moved to a bed and lay down. I opened her suicide gown and was shocked at the number of scratch marks on her chest and abdomen. Some of them were six inches in length. I began cleaning each of them and dressing them as best as possible, with her being on suicide watch.

I asked, "What exactly happened last night?"

"I was attacked…as I always am."

"Any history of drug use?"

"Everyone always asks this."

"And?"

"I haven't used drugs in years. I only used meth a little and some marijuana."

"None recently and certainly none since I came to prison."

"How long have you been in prison?"

"Two years, and I have three more to go." Desri was both angry and frustrated. It showed in her protective arms across her chest and in her voice."

"When did you first notice these bugs on your skin?"

"Don't know."

"Do you see them now?"

"Heck no. They only come out at night. It's like they're sleeping during the day."

"What kind of bugs do you see?"

Desri shivered. Some can be long with tons of legs. Others are like ants. They are disgusting. I don't know why they like to live in my skin."

Twenty minutes later, I was finished addressing her wounds.

"What's going to happen to me?" asked Desri. "Are you going to stick me back into the cell so they can attack me again? Still think I want to hurt myself?"

"I'm going to talk with the doctor and see if we can help you." I walked out, and it took a few minutes to find the physician. I explained to him everything I had seen since Desri arrived. He listened and began nodding part way through my explanation. He agreed to join me in medical and talk with Desri.

Stepping inside the exam room, Desri became withdrawn and began denying anything had ever happened to her. She denied any thoughts or ideas of seeing bugs.

Dr. Dewey said, "I've actually seen a few patients who saw bugs before. It isn't real common, but it's happened before."

"That's not me. I don't know what Nurse Campbell told you, but it isn't true. She's trying to convince you that I'm sick in the mind. Another excuse to keep me locked up in solitary."

"I don't think so," said Dr. Dewey.

Desri peered at me and said, "She trippin'. I'm fine."

"Hear me out. It usually happens in one of two ways. First, you hear from someone else a story about a spider or something in their cell or maybe their house. You hate how the story sounds and how it makes you feel. Many people have phobias of bugs. You then start thinking about what would happen if that occurred to you. Soon enough, you can't stop thinking and dreaming about bugs."

Desir interrupted, "No one told me no stories." Her face had gone pale.

"The second possibility is that you see an actual spider or a bug on you. You knock it away, and it comes back over and over again. Soon, you have bugs approaching all the time, especially at night. They might come from the corners of the room or from right under your skin."

"Stop!" screamed Desri. "I don't want to talk about this."

"Fine," said Dr. Dewey. "I just want you to know there is treatment for this. We can help you."

"No thanks. I want to go back to my cell...now!"

I said, "I'll stop by in a few days to check on you."

"Don't bother," replied Desri. She was returned to her cell, and I didn't see her for a few days.

My time off was just what I needed. Working in a prison can be difficult and draining. But I was also excited to return back. Dr. Dewey found me within ten minutes of clocking in. He had a smile on his face.

"What's going on?" I asked.

"Desri Stevens finally agreed to treatment. We've started her on medications, and she's been doing well the last few nights. She's also working with mental health to get through a few things."

"That's a great thing."

He leaned closer. "It got awful the next two nights after we talked to her. The scratches were worse the first night. The second night she slammed her head into the wall."

"No way."

"She nearly knocked herself unconscious."

"Was she really seeing bugs?"

"In her mind, yes. It is called Formication. It can be real to her."

"What is it caused by?"

"Trauma, mental health, drug use, fear, or even phobia. You name it. I just hope she is willing to take her medications going forward."

"Can she get rid of it?"

"Maybe. It'll take a lot of therapy and dealing with things. Medications can help too."

I said, "That was one of the craziest things I've ever seen."

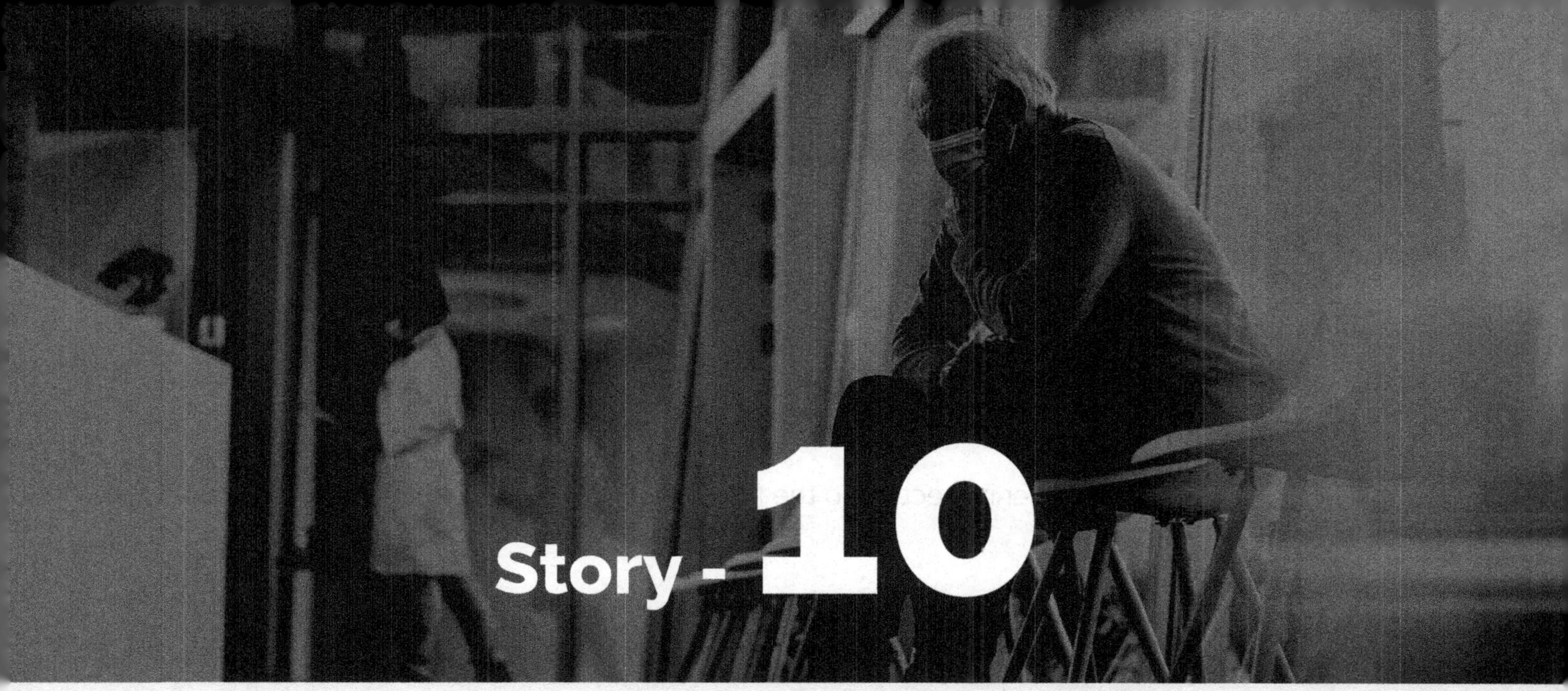

Story - 10

Consequence of Leaving the Hospital Against Medical Advice

A fifty-one year old man was found unconscious in Radcliff Park with slow breathing, an elevated blood sugar above 500, and other injuries, and despite the paramedic's attempts, they could not wake him. The ambulance transported him to the closest hospital, and an IV was started en route. Dr. Babington was prepped, and his team was ready for the arrival of the unconscious patient.

The ambulance pulled up to the outer bay of the hospital, and the man was moved quickly inside and into a trauma room. He had active bleeding on the forehead, cuts on both arms and blood stained down his left leg. Initially, it was hard to tell what had happened to him and how much damage there was.

The first responders worried it might have been from an attack, and the wounds were consistent with this type of injury. The patient had an ID and was found to be Mr. Fomina.

Dr. Babington said, "Check the head and neck for any open wounds or other signs of head trauma."

Nurse Blye Vernon said, "Looks clean. There are some old scrapes, but nothing new, except the laceration to the forehead."

"What about pupil reaction?"

"They're round and equal seized. They react normally."

"Good. We might need to order a head CT just to make sure," replied Dr. Babington.

Nurse Blye nodded and moved her inspection to the forehead. She began to clean the wound to see how deep it was.

"We've got some puncture marks," said Nurse Jonathan Smiley as he worked on the left arm. "If I had to guess, probably some bites from a dog."

"Let's start an antibiotic," said Dr. Babington. "Are the bites fresh or old?"

"Fresh."

Dr. Babington began pressing on the chest and abdomen. He listened to the lungs. "What is his blood sugar?"

A third nurse, Bobbie Armstead, said, "Still in the 500's."

Start an Insulin drip," said Dr. Babington. We need to get his blood sugars more under control. Has anyone looked at his lower legs?"

"On it," said Nurse Blye. A few minutes later, she said, "He has a pressure ulcer on the bottom of his left foot. He has had two of his toes amputated on his right foot."

"Is this guy in our system?"

An ancillary staff standing near the door said, "He's been here twice before. A year ago and three years ago. We have him listed as homeless, a veteran, who has been going to the homeless clinic on 53rd Street for his medications. He has been on Insulin for over ten years."

"What did we see him for last time?"

"Intoxication and Pneumonia the most recent time. Before that, it was for Diabetic Ketoacidosis, and both times he stayed overnight. He had an ambulation of his toes three years ago."

"Well," said Dr. Babington. "It looks like he was attacked. He has injuries consistent with being punched and/or kicked. I'm not sure how the dog fits into this. Let's get him some fluids, Chest X-ray, and a head CT. Right now, he is stable, but we need that blood sugar down. Let's order some STAT labs and we need to get a urine. We can cath him if needed. Let me know if he becomes unstable.

The three nurses nodded and got to work. The fluids were already running, and setting up an Insulin drip was easy. Within twenty minutes, his blood sugars were starting to improve. During that time, they cathed him and got a sample of blood to be sent for testing. The urine was dark, almost amber in color. There wasn't a lot they were able to get. They placed an indwelling Foley catheter to remain in his bladder and collect urine continually. Next, they sent him first for the head CT. This was followed by a chest X-ray.

The chest X-ray showed pneumonia, and antibiotics were started. Within an hour, several things had happened. He had been ruled out of anything alarming in the brain, such as significant head trauma, stroke, or brain bleed. He was started on antibiotics both for the bite and the pneumonia. He had no broken bones but was in Ketoacidosis, a condition of high blood sugar without proper treatment.

Dr. Babington was pleased with the findings and was hopeful that the patient would start to improve. Mr. Fomina made a turn for the better a short time later. His blood sugars and urine color improved, and the treatment was starting to work.

When Mr. Fomina woke up, however, he was in a panic. He started screaming and thrashing and nearly ripped his IV and Insulin drip from his arm. He was crazed, speaking incoherently and yelling that something was missing. The staff tried to control him, but it wasn't working. At some point, he was given an injection to rest.

A few hours later, he woke up far calmer and more relaxed. The treatments provided were really starting to improve his conditions. He was less pale, and his injuries were bandaged. He was hungry and less paranoid.

Dr. Babington came in as soon as he could. He asked, "Mr. Fomina, how are you feeling?"

"When can I get out of here?" Mr. Fomina was eating a sandwich.

"We have a few more tests to run, but you're doing much better. Your blood sugars have been stable in the last hour or so. We need to get more fluids into you."

"I'm fine, doctor. I just need to leave here."

"What is the rush?"

"You wouldn't understand."

"It looks like you were attacked, and your blood sugar was really elevated."

"I can't afford medications such as Insulin. I'm doing the best that I can. That's not what is important right now."

Mr. Fomina was beginning to get agitated again.

Dr. Babington asked, "What is the most important thing for you?"

"Finding my dog. Someone tried stealing him."

"Is that where you got those dog bites?"

"Someone came to take him. I was trying to get him back. I was hit and kicked, but they were stealing my dog."

"Who?"

"It doesn't matter. You wouldn't believe me."

Dr. Babington asked, "Who?"

"It was the government. They are using my dog to spy on me."

"I see," said Dr. Babington. "I'm going to call in the nurse, and we can try to help you."

"I want to leave. Right now!!" Mr. Fomina began screaming again. "I know my rights. You can't hold me. I want to leave AMA."

"Raising two hands, Dr. Babington asked, "You want to leave against medical advice. That doesn't have to happen."

"I need to find my dog." In one quick swipe, he pulled out his IV. Glancing down at the Foley Cath, he said, "You can remove this, or I will."

"Fine," said Dr. Babington. "I will call in a nurse, and we can prepare your things."

"Thank you. I just need to find my dog."

Mr. Fomina signed the AMA and was discharged from the hospital. He left with a script for Insulin, antibiotics, and a referral to a shelter near 47th Street, not far from where he was found.

Two weeks later, he was brought back to the hospital with symptoms similar to before. His blood sugars were sky-high, and he hadn't showered in weeks. The infection in his arm had gone untreated, and his skin was red and irritated. This time, he hadn't been assaulted, but he had lost more than ten pounds of weight. He looked far worse than before.

This time, it took nearly two days for the IV fluids, medications, and Insulin to bring Mr. Fomina into a steady state. He was sick, pale, and uncomfortable, and the ulcers on his feet had worsened dramatically. It was obvious he wasn't feeling very well.

It was an entirely different staff at the hospital that day, except for one nurse, but they were able to review the chart, and the treatment again was initiated. They gave fluids and IV antibiotics to help with the infection. When he awoke and could answer questions, they had a plan in place. They had a social worker available and had contacted a shelter and a local agency that could provide some of his diabetic medications.

Mr. Fomina didn't care. He was beside himself. "I just need to find my dog."

The doctor said, "We have someone willing to call all the animal shelters. We will help you look for your dog if you stay here for treatment. Just give us his name and a picture or a description. We will do everything we can to help."

This caused Mr. Fomina to pause and consider their proposal. After thinking about it for a few minutes, he nodded and sat back to rest. More fluids were ordered, blood work tested, and they scheduled a shower in fifteen minutes. Afterward, they would bandage his feet.

Mr. Fomina was calm, and when the social worker came in, he could describe the dog, a mixed golden retriever named Rosco. It turned out that the government hadn't stolen his dog, but rather another homeless man who had been attacked a few times wanted Mr. Fomina's dog for protection. The two had fought. His dog had accidentally bitten him when he was getting taken. When Mr. Fomina was released the last time, he couldn't track down the guy who stole his dog.

Nurse Jonathan came in and removed the line to his IV. A dressing was placed over the area so he could shower. Mr. Fomina was escorted to the shower and given some privacy.

They knocked on the door when he didn't come out after fifteen minutes. There was no answer. They called the charge nurse and were given permission to enter the room. Nurse Jonathan was given a key, and he and another nurse went in. The shower was still on, but Mr. Fomina had vanished out a back door. The hospital was searched, but Mr. Fomina was gone.

Despite their best efforts, the patient had chosen to leave the hospital. Sometimes we are our own worst enemies.

Three days later, the ambulance was called to Radcliff Park for an unconscious male. By the time the paramedic arrived, the man had passed away. Statements were taken, and many of the workers in the area recognized the guy. He would go day and night, screaming and searching for his dog. It was heartbreaking for the paramedics and hospital staff to learn what happened to Mr. Fomina. He had been so fixated on finding his dog that he refused to take care of himself, and ultimately it cost him his life.

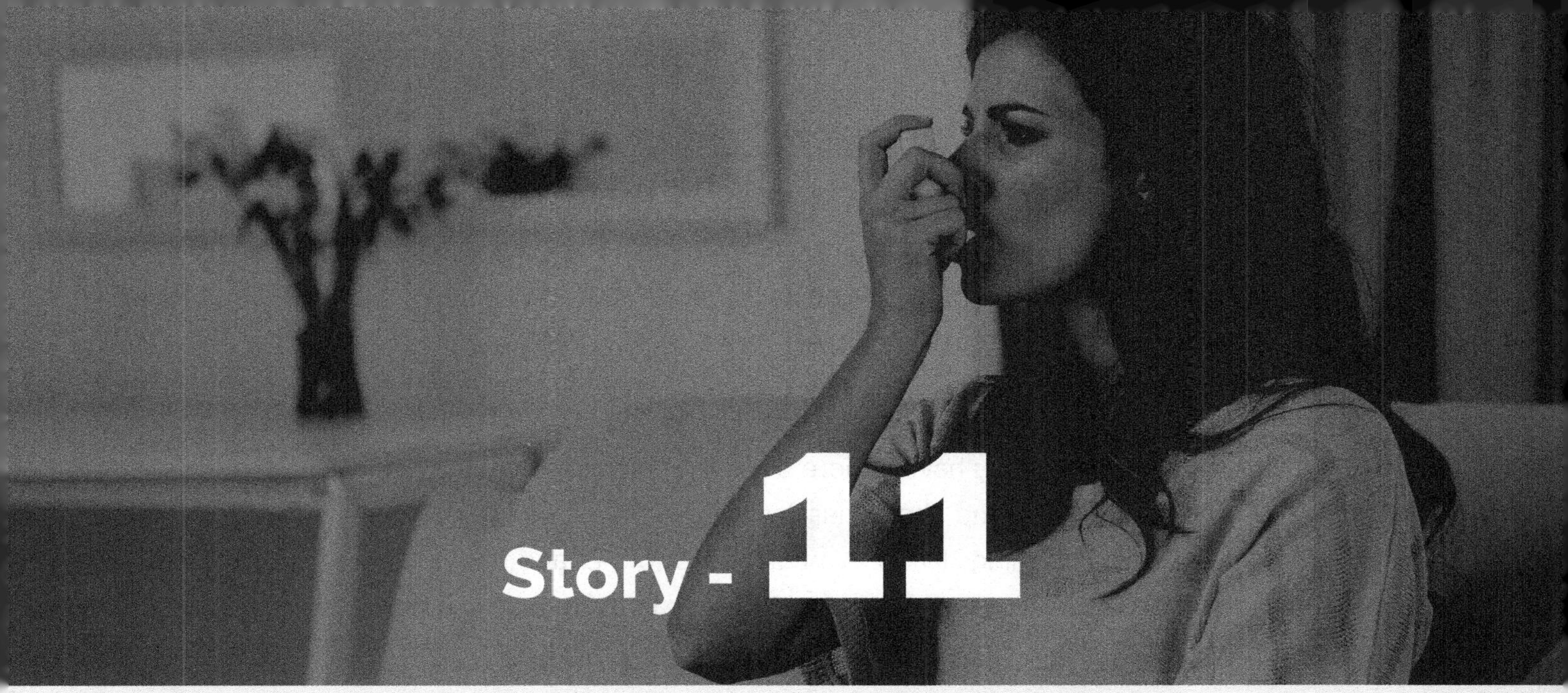

Story - 11

Triggers of an Asthma Exacerbation

Our respiratory department is attached to a hospital and the Emergency Room. This means we have patients who come in for routine exams to our offices and follow-ups. Other times, we're called to the ER at all times of the day for emergencies involving the Respiratory process. Some of these patients are fixed at the moment, and others require further assessments over the next subsequent weeks.

A young girl around ten had been to the hospital approximately three times before our department was called in to help. She was diagnosed through her pediatrician about a year before in connection with exercise and cold weather. She was ordered an inhaler very sparingly. It didn't seem to us that she was using her inhaler correctly, but we didn't come to this conclusion until after someone called the fourth time.

Chart records show the first three ER visits were for asthma exacerbations. Rebecca Caldwell would come in to get treatment at the ER. She would often get a nebulizer treatment and some steroids. She received an antibiotic once because the ER staff was worried an infection might be involved. All three times, the severity of the attack was about the same, mild-to-moderate. She was not kept overnight.

After the third visit, the ER doctor talked with my colleague and me to ensure that everything was done right. It was, and I told him that we would have done the same thing. We gave some recommendations for him to consider if she came in a fourth time. Fast forward six months and Rebecca was returning to the ER with difficulty breathing. This time we were notified immediately.

When my team arrived, Rebecca was having more trouble than usual, catching her breath. She was sitting awkwardly and using all her neck and chest muscles to try to slow and deepen her breathing. It looked like she had been taught some things to do. We felt so sad for her and the stress it was causing her and her family. It's accurate to say that someone going through an asthma attack feels like they are trying to suck air through a straw.

Rebecca had just played a soccer game, gone home, and two hours later, her home inhalers were not helping her wheezing. From there, her parents tried to shower her with no luck. They were forced to call an ambulance.

We immediately started her on oxygen, and this only helped minimally. A nebulizer treatment was started through the same mask giving oxygen, and it took two treatments, but the look on her face when she finally started breathing better was precious. It's always a relief to see the patient improving and starting to recover.

Rebecca was admitted overnight and through most of the next day. Early the following morning, she didn't require oxygen when sitting and only when going to the bathroom or walking around the unit. By the afternoon, she didn't require oxygen at all.

Before she was released, I asked, "Did you play your soccer game outside?"

"Yes. On grass."

"Did you see a lot of pollen?"

"None at all. The grass didn't seem to bother me. The game was super cold and rainy. It was the coldest game of the season."

"Did you use your inhaler before the game?"

"No," she answered.

I said, "For the next several games, try using your inhaler before the games, even if you don't feel any chest tightness or wheezing."

"Okay."

I gave the same recommendation to both parents. I also scheduled a follow-up visit in two weeks in my office and recommended that Rebecca used an air humidifier in her room when she slept. The parents insisted that they would get one right away. Two weeks later, Rebecca came in and said that she was doing well. During her last two soccer games, she had no problems breathing. At home, she felt great.

"Great," I said.

"Thank you, doctor Maddison. I think we might have turned a corner."

I saw Rebecca a month later, three months later, and all seemed great.

But just six months later, Rebecca was brought back to the ER with a severe asthma attack. As before, this time was worse than the previous one. She arrived already on oxygen and was unconscious, barely breathing. It took the ER staff and the Respiratory staff quite some time before she was stable. She stayed in the hospital for three days during this hospitalization. New medications were added, and she left feeling great. However, I was worried that something more was going on that I couldn't see.

I spoke with the parents on our subsequent visit without Rebecca in the room about allergies, other medications, and consistency with treatment. The parents explained that Rebecca was almost religious when it came to taking her medications. They had no pets and had no plans of getting any. She had some allergies, but not to food and primarily to pollen or grass. But her asthma never got this bad when she was around those things.

Two weeks later, she was back in the ER. This time, a ventilator was required, which meant that a breathing machine was used. She remained hooked up to the ventilator for three days. She was on oxygen for another two days after the tube was removed.

The day before she was to be released, Rebecca became quite warm in her room. This wasn't because of a sickness or anything related to her condition. She asked if the window could be opened. One of my therapists was slightly worried the cold air might be causing her problems. A chart review showed that almost all her asthma problems had occurred in the winter.

The therapist opened the window slightly, and the cold air rushed into the room. Rebecca kept breathing without a single problem or change for the first fifteen minutes. The therapist and staff were prepared if something changed. After fifteen minutes, it did...but it wasn't from the cold. A waft of smoke from a cigarette came in through the window, and Rebecca reacted to it immediately.

She started coughing, choking, and wheezing. The window was closed, oxygen was placed on her face, and it took thirty minutes for her lungs to calm down. The Respiratory Therapist contacted me immediately. and I came to talk with Mom and Dad.

The parents admitted that they smoke inside the house, but usually the windows are open during the summer and closed during the winter. There have been times that they try to smoke outside, but it has become a habit to smoke inside.

I explained, "It has become clear to my staff and me that Rebecca is highly reactionary to smoking. This doesn't happen to everyone who has asthma and is around smoke. Asthma can have many triggers, and I think smoke is Rebecca's trigger. Her lungs start having airway contractions, and she has an asthma execration."

They asked, "Can we smoke outside?"

"No. You'll need to quit. The smoke will linger on your clothes. Even keeping the windows open won't help. Rebecca is getting more and more sensitive to smoke. The next time could be much worse."

The parents agreed to quit, and a few days later, Rebecca was discharged from the hospital.

Six months later, Rebecca was twelve and returned to the ER unconscious and not breathing. The parents were beside themselves. Luckily, Rebecca responded to oxygen and treatment and didn't require intubation.

I spoke with the ambulance crew, and they confirmed my suspicions. The parent's house was filled with smoke. They had bought a humidifier and placed it in Rebecca's room. The windows were open when the paramedics arrived, but the amount of smoke inside the house was toxic.

After treating Rebecca, the hospitalist, myself, the ER doctor, and Social Services went into a room with the parents and spoke with them as sternly as possible.

"If you don't stop smoking, you will end up killing Rebecca. I am tempted to ask social services to intervene and remove Rebecca from your house."

"Please don't do that," the parents cried. "We can change."

"Rebecca's risk was clear the last time we spoke."

"We tried opening the windows and getting a humidifier."

"That was not the recommendation," I protested. "You cannot continue to smoke. Even if you do it far away from Rebecca, she will smell it when you get back, even if you can't."

"We will do better," they promised.

A contract was signed, and social services informed the family that they would come to the family's home to check on them.

The parents agreed.

I heard sometime later that Rebecca went to live with the mother's sister for a few months as the parents worked through quitting. In the end, they did quit smoking, and Rebecca became acutely aware of the dangers of smoke. As time went on, her reaction to smoke lessened as long as she wasn't around it a lot. However, if her parents started smoking again, she would not be able to live with them. It was that severe and dangerous.

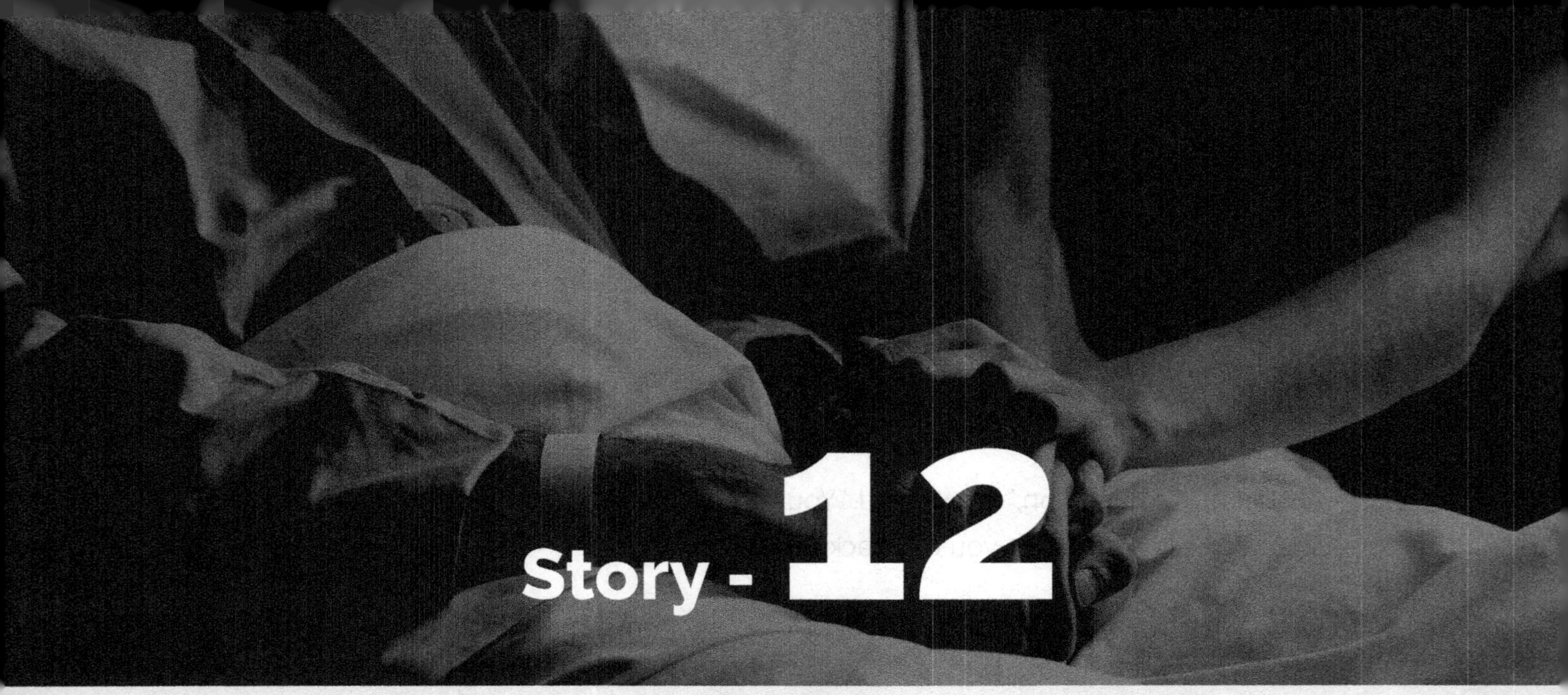

Story - 12

When the Deep Freeze Isn't a Terrible Thing

Chad Barlow played professional basketball overseas for five years after going undrafted. He loved each and every minute. But by the time he'd finished his fifth season, though, he and his wife had three children, and it was time to come back home to the states.

Life happened. He got a regular job, grew older, and watched his children. But he never stopped playing basketball. He joined some competitive leagues with other players who had played in college. But over time, he got slower and couldn't jump quite as well. But that didn't stop him.

When Chad was in his mid-forties, he was playing for a competitive rec league with seven other players. They had played together for five years, except for one player that was added the year before. They knew each other well and their families and were having a lot of fun. They won most of their games but lost plenty too.

The fourth game of the weekend was going better than Chad had expected. He was running up and down the court, hitting shots, and felt like he was getting his legs back after a cold two weeks before. During the third quarter, however, he felt suddenly like he had lost the ability to breathe. His team called a time-out, and he was helped to the bench. Initially, it was thought that he needed a few minutes to catch his breath. The new guy, Ted, jumped in, and the game continued. Chad slumped to the floor two minutes later, and the entire team rushed forward.

Ted cried, "Someone, call an ambulance."

"Does anyone know where the AED is?" asked the team's coach.

"I do," said someone from the stands.

The AED, or automated external defibrillator, was immediately brought over to where Chad lay on the court. Other players, including Ted, had checked for a pulse, and after finding none, started CPR. Chest compressions were continued until the AED was set into place.

Lisa, Chad's wife, rushed over hysterically. "What's happening?" she demanded.

"Chad isn't breathing," a friend explained. "They called an ambulance and started CPR. He might have had a heart attack."

"I can't believe this is happening," said Lisa.

Those helping with the situation followed the directions on the AED and placed pads directly on Chad's chest. The AED analyzed the heart rhythm and determined that a shock was advised.

The AED delivered a shock, but nothing happened. The heart didn't start, and there was still no pulse. CPR was started again.

Lisa asked, "What does that mean?"

"We need the ambulance to get here as soon as possible," said the coach.

The ambulance arrived only a few minutes later. Paramedics ran in, assessed the scene, and knew that Chad needed to be transported. He was transferred into their care and onto a gurney, all while CPR continued. An IV was placed in his arm, and medications were given.

On the ride to the hospital, Chad was shocked two more times. CPR continued for the entire time. Approximately twenty-eight minutes after Chad initially went down, the paramedics felt a faint pulse. This was a good thing, but there were still plenty of things that needed to be done.

At the hospital, the emergency room staff and cardiologist were ready for his arrival. Chad was brought into the hospital room and immediately underwent assessment and evaluation. It took an hour to get testing done, blood work, and an angiogram of the heart. This scan looks at the blood flow going in and out of the heart, including arteries or veins. Often heart blocks are seen. It helps to know if a stent needs to be placed. Without oxygen, the tissue of the heart or brain can be damaged. Other parts of the body are affected as well.

Chad was finally stabilized but did not wake up and was in a coma. When someone is in this situation, after having suffered cardiac arrest, they're much more likely to have another heart attack or a stroke. Chad was placed on several medications and transferred to a portion of the hospital where he could be monitored.

Family and friends arrived to see how Chad was doing. His coach, teammates, and family were in shock. It became quickly known that Chad didn't have a personal or family history of cardiac problems. He wasn't taking any medications that would put him at risk or were used to treat a cardiac history.

Doctor Filmore came to Chad's wife, Lisa, and their children and explained the risks and the possible outcomes. Although Chad was stable, he wasn't out of the woods by any means. Additionally, they couldn't predict how Chad would be if and when he recovered.

On the second day of his coma, it was decided that Chad needed additional and more advanced treatment. There was no way to know how he would be affected by the lack of oxygenated blood going to his brain. It was good that he received CPR so quickly, but Doctor Filmore and others decided that Chad would undergo Therapeutic Hypothermia.

Doctor Filmore explained to Chad's wife the benefits of this treatment. She agreed immediately for them to proceed.

Therapeutic Hypothermia pushes Chad's temperature to 92 degrees. It's attempting to help Chad's brain and prevent any further damage. Over the next few days, Chad received this treatment and was given IV fluids, electrolytes, and additional medications.

A brain scan showed that Chad's brain had some swelling. This was likely from the initial cardiac event and some of the treatment he received. By dropping the temperature, the doctors were hopeful it would reverse the swelling and reduce the risk factors for seizures and other problems.

Chad awoke from his coma on the tenth day. His wife and one of his children were in the room.

"Where am I?" asked Chad. He glanced around the hospital room as if he'd been on a different planet. Lisa and his son rushed forward to calm Chad.

"At the hospital," replied Lisa. "You're going to be fine."

"What happened?"

"You had a heart attack on the court."

"Are you joking?"

Lisa was crying. She couldn't say anything, but she started to cry.

Ricky, their middle child, explained what happened as Doctor Filmore was called for a full assessment.

Dr. Filmore asked, "What do you remember?"

"I ate oatmeal, bacon, and eggs for breakfast," said Chad.

Dr. Filmore laughed. In truth, Chad suffered some significant memory loss. But as Dr. Filmore explained, "It's great that he can talk, move his extremities, and remember some of what happened. A slight memory problem isn't unexpected."

"What happened to me?" asked Chad an hour later. Lisa had to explain everything all over again.

"Can I play basketball again?" asked Chad.

Dr. Filmore said, "We really don't know. You've done far better than we could have hoped. You didn't have a pulse for almost thirty minutes. That often means that we don't expect quite as good of an outcome."

"But what about basketball?"

"It all depends on how your body reacts to treatment and therapy, and it will take time to understand what, if any, damage there was to your heart."

"What other problems could I have?"

"Many," said Dr. Filmore. "In truth, if this was five or ten years ago, you probably wouldn't have survived. The Therapeutic Hypothermia was a game changer for you. We preserved your tissues by lowering your temperature. It was a miracle."

Chad was released from the hospital ten days later. He had a dozen new medications but was told that if things progressed, he would get off most of them. He had significant memory issues for several months and even longer. One of the unique things was that he couldn't remember the name of his youngest daughter for the longest time. He left the hospital in a wheelchair, though he was encouraged to walk as much as possible. He had trouble flexing and extending his left foot for almost a year and had to wear a brace. It only slightly affected his walk.

Today, Chad is doing well. He loves to shoot the basket, but he will never play in a competitive league again. He has his heart checked out every six months. He takes his medications and feels lucky to have survived his heart attack.

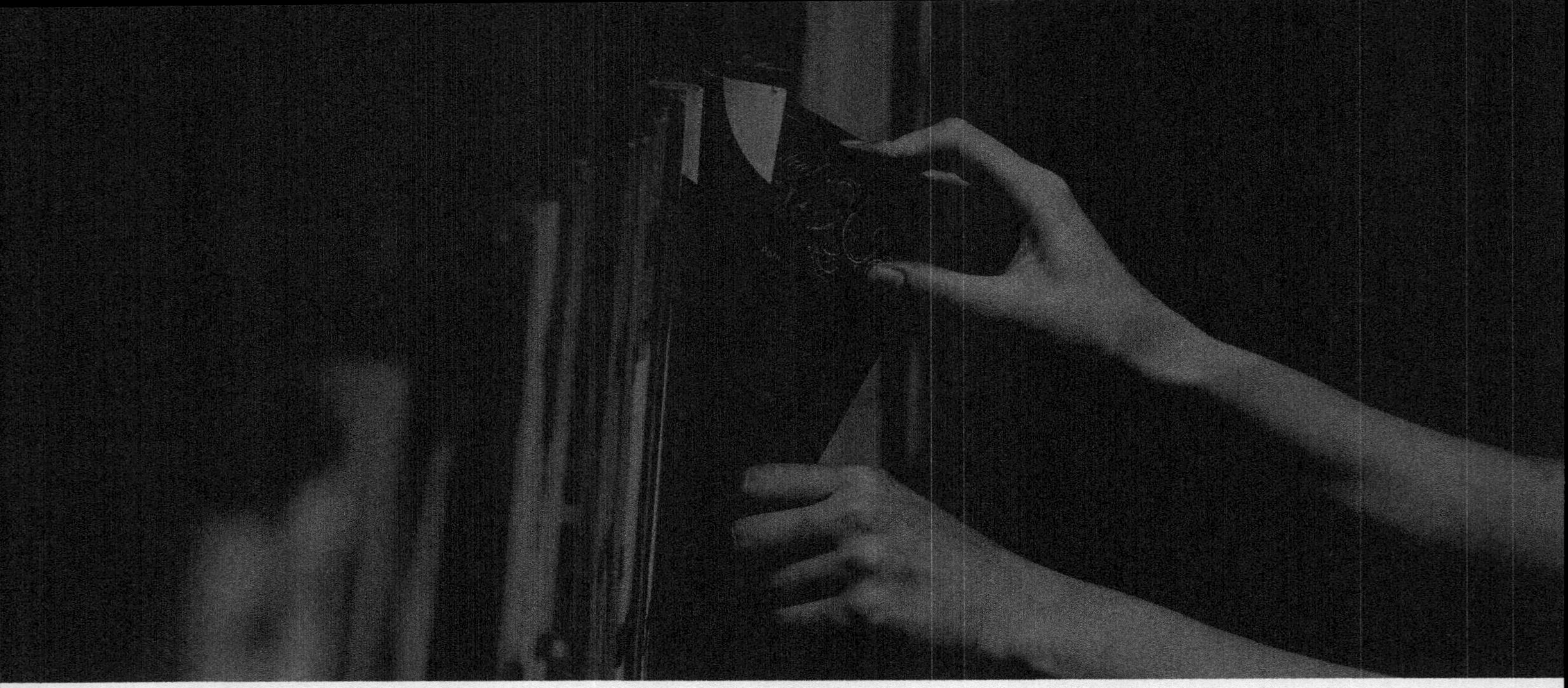

Tales of the Exam Room Collection

***Crazy Medical Stories:* Tales of the Exam Room Volume 1**

10 Short stories about the crazy world of Medicine. These stories have taken years to collect, understand, and write. Author Scott Kemp has worked tirelessly to bring for you this entertaining perspective of the patient and medical staff relationship. Each story brings about a greater clarity into the delicate choices presented day in and day out.

https://www.amazon.com/Crazy-Medical-Stories-Tales-Exam/dp/1736159844/ref=tmm_pap_swatch_0?_encoding=UTF8&qid=1618501286&sr=8-2

***Medical Horror Stories:* Tales of the Exam Room Volume 2**

10 Short stories about the crazy world of Medicine. In Vol 2, we continue exploring the astonishing world of medicine as we discover some of the unpredictable situations between patients and medical professionals. Often, like a law of nature, when something can go wrong, it does. But the outcome is rarely as you expect it.

https://www.amazon.com/Medical-Horror-Stories-Tales-Exam/dp/1736159860/ref=sr_1_5?dchild=1&keywords=Tales+of+the+Exam+room&qid=1613685694&sr=8-5

***Medical Stories While Incarcerated:* Tales of the Exam Room Volume 3**

12 Short stories about the crazy world of Medicine. Medicine happens in all shapes and forms. We are excited to present these stories centered around medical stories that happen in jails and prisons. But beware, these stories are a step or two more graphic than our previous stories. We have a long-standing love for medicine and some of the unimaginable situations that patients and medical professionals find themselves in.

https://www.amazon.com/Tales-Exam-Room-Medical-Incarcerated/dp/B08NYTQ6GX/ref=sr_1_4?dchild=1&keywords=Tales+of+the+Exam+Room&qid=1606499209&sr=8-4

***Scary Medical Stories:* Tales of the Exam Room Volume 4**

12 Short stories in Vol. 4 that takes a look into the extreme side of medicine. This includes a boy getting hit in the chest with a ball, relenting episodes of vomiting, and much more. This set of stories helps you appreciate the importance and impact of medical professionals in difficult situations.

Scary Medical Stories: Tales of the Exam Room Volume 4: Kemp, Scott: 9781954814059: Amazon.com: Books

***Amusing Medical Stories:* Tales of the Exam Room Volume 5**

12 Short stories in Vol. 5 has stories that are intended to be felt, enjoyed, and told repeatedly. There is so much to learn about patient encounters, decision-making disasters, and the incredible actions of those involved during odd and life-saving situations. This certainly doesn't mean that each story will have a happy ending.

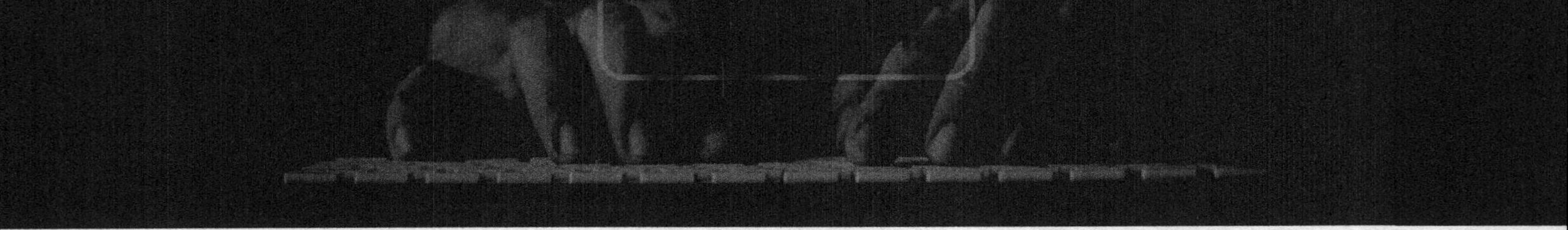

Sign up for our Newsletter

Join us @ Exam Room Tales to get a better look at what we do. We will also offer special promos, and you will receive benefits for signing up for our newsletter. Our team sends out a Newsletter several times a year.

The goal of the Newsletter is to keep our readers up to date on what we are working on. It also offers a platform to provide feedback, share stories, and much more. Our Newsletter team will also offer promos, special offers, incentives, unique stories, and more.

Come Join us ExamRoomTales.com

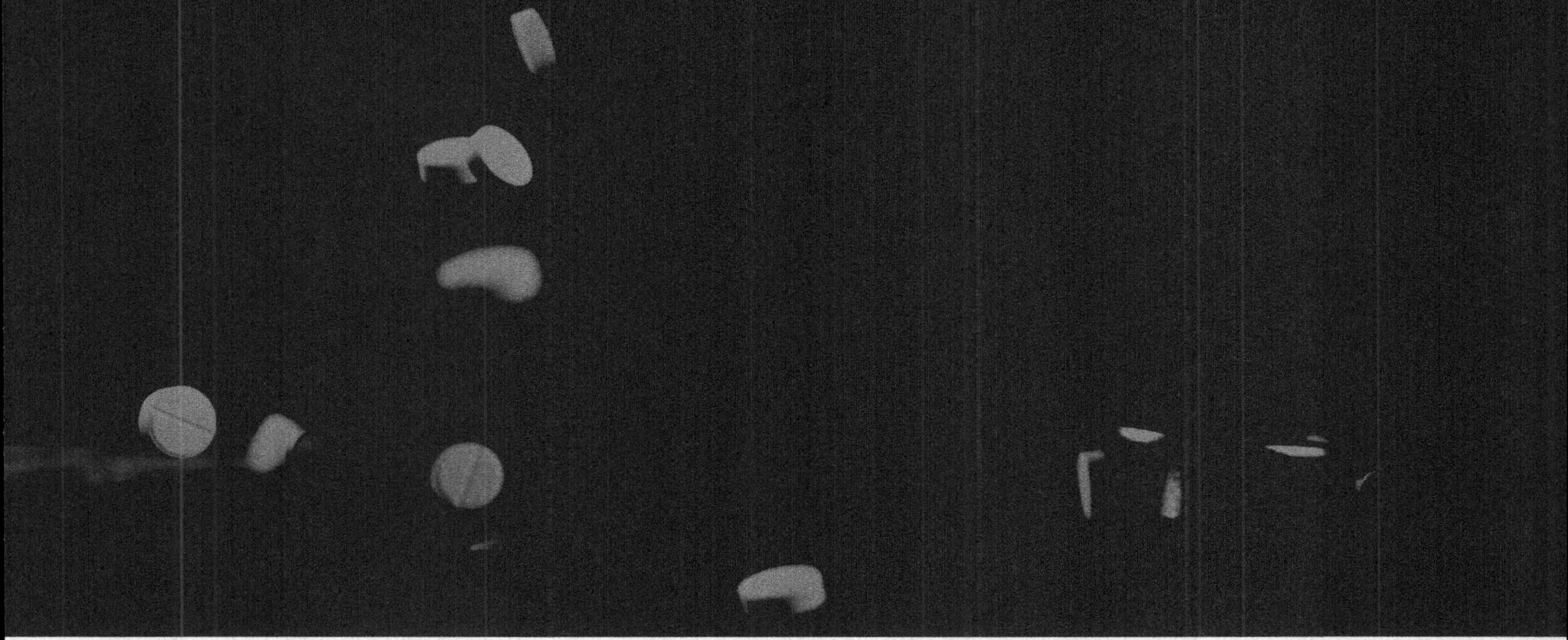

Background on Correctional Medicine in the United States

Many of our tales come from the world of prisons and jails. This is a general information sheet that we include in all our volumes. If you've read it before, please move on. However, the message is still important.

The United States has, by far, one of the highest rates of incarceration in the world. As of 2016 – 655 inmates per 100,000 are found within the jails and prisons of America. But other countries around the world are also experiencing an increase in the number of individuals incarcerated. Many different countries have tried different things to curb incarceration rates – some work, and some do not.

Each country has specific and unique ways to handle the medical needs required for inmates. This need may be overlooked or misunderstood by the general public when dealing with cost, workforce, funding, and many other areas of correctional responsibilities.

Additionally, millions of individuals have been freed from jails and prisons that are being monitored on probation or parole. This also adds to the responsibilities of the government, cities, towns, and communities. For those younger than 18 – there are often detention centers.

Correctional Medicine is challenging and unique. Inmates can be difficult to treat for several reasons, including risk factors, past medical histories, unique circumstances, unique mental health problems, difficulty following directions, homelessness, and many others. This isn't to say that every inmate falls into the category of being difficult. For some reason, the most unexpected things happen in prisons and jails.

Constitutionally, inmates should be provided with reasonable medical and mental health care. That means you can't lock them up and throw away the key. Many times, there are dental issues, pending surgeries, medications, serious medical and mental health conditions, and many more circumstances that should be considered and often continued if possible.

Not all medications that a patient takes on the streets will be allowed in a correctional facility. There are hundreds of different prisons and jails throughout the United States. This includes Federal prison/jails, state prisons, and many other forms of detention centers. Each facility will do things a little differently from one to another. This could be based on region, size, beliefs, medical knowledge, medical personnel, administration, financial, and many other things. In essence, what works for one jail may not work for another.

The medicine inside correctional facilities can be exciting, difficult, and even disturbing. It is rare when someone is satisfied with the level of care they are receiving, even if it is exceeding the standards available. Lawsuits are often brought against medical personnel, prisons, and jails. Some of these are for a good reason, but many are not.

The truth of the matter is that inmates are people and should be treated with appropriate medical care regardless of the crimes that brought them to the correctional facilities. On the opposite side of the coin, the medical staff is often attacked, berated, threatened, and more when they are trying to do the best job they can.

The following stories are intended to give the reader a picture into some of the crazier and unbelievable aspects of medicine. These stories are based on true situations, but many things have been changed to protect the patient. Some stories have been combined or changed to give the reader a better understanding and picture of the world of correction medicine.

To our knowledge, all patients involved received excellent health care.

Please enjoy!!

Made in the USA
Monee, IL
08 November 2026

67948337R00044